GREEN CLEAN YOUR HOME

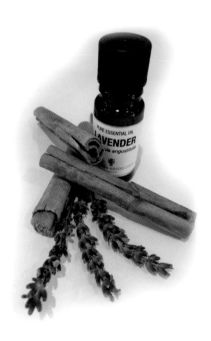

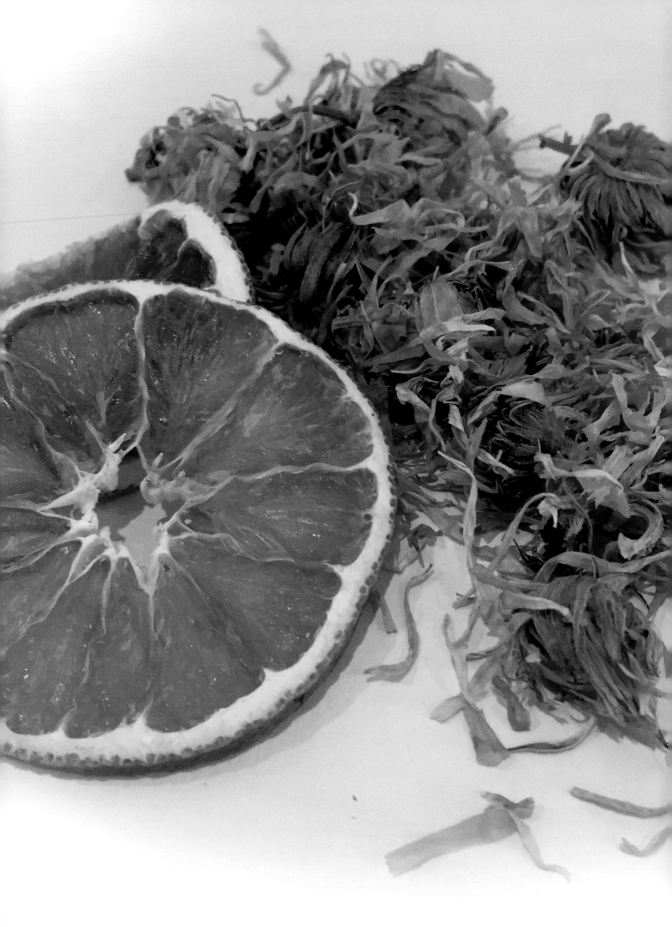

GREEN CLEAN
YOUR HOME

160 simple, nature-friendly
recipes which really work

Manfred Neuhold

MERLIN UNWIN BOOKS

This edition published in Great Britain by Merlin Unwin Books, 2020
First published in Germany by L.V. Buch, Munster 2017

Merlin Unwin Books Ltd
Palmers House
7 Corve Street
Ludlow
Shropshire SY8 1DB
UK

www.merlinunwin.co.uk

Designed and typeset in 12 point Minion Pro by Jo Dovey
Science consultant Andrew Moss

Printed by Star Standard Industries (PTE) Ltd

*Photographs on pages 11, 26, 88, 134, 150, 174, 184 and on front and back
cover are reproduced under license from Shutterstock.com

CONTENTS

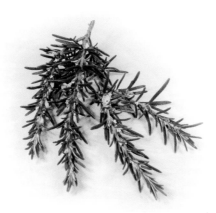

GLOSSARY

The word in bold below is the term we have used throughout the book for the following synonyms.

Caustic soda: sodium hydroxide, lye

Washing soda: sodium carbonate, soda crystals, soda powder

Bicarbonate of soda: baking soda, sodium bicarbonate

Cream of tartar: tartaric acid

Baking powder: cream of tartar mixed with bicarbonate of soda

Surfactant: a wetting agent, or tenside, one which reduces the surface tension. If coconut-derived, it is a coconut surfactant or tenside

OCCASIONAL MINOR ADJUSTMENTS TO SUIT YOURSELF

The environmentally-friendly products that you will buy to make the recipes in this book may vary slightly from shop to shop and manufacturer to manufacturer. With the exception of the soap-making on pages 202-203, don't be afraid to add a little more, or sometimes less, water to your recipe to obtain the right consistency. It will not compromise the effectiveness of your finished product. You will quickly learn the exact proportions through experimentation.

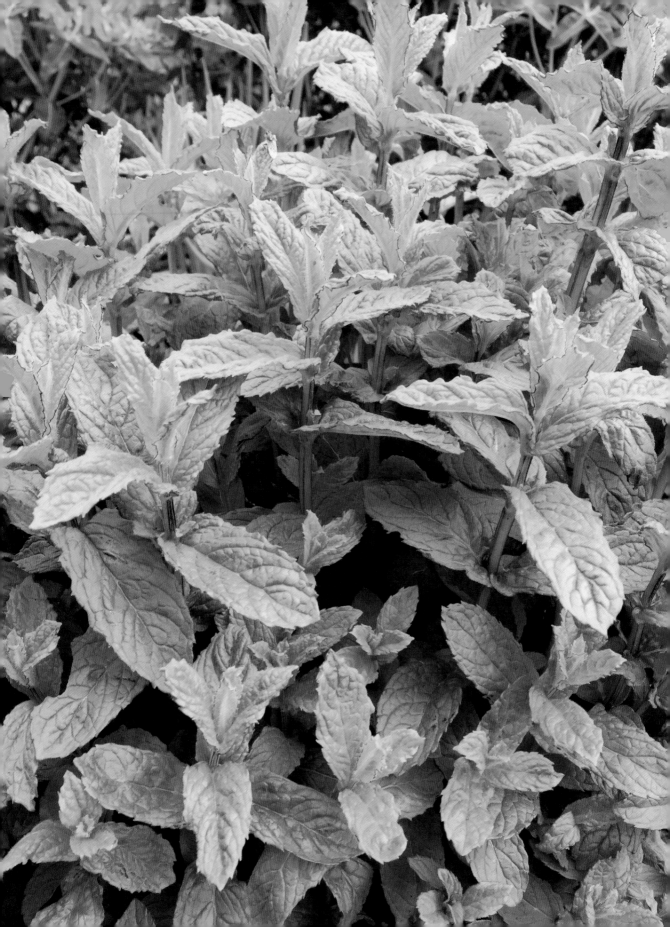

CHAPTER ONE

THE SHORT PHILOSOPHY OF CLEANING

KEEPING YOUR OWN ENVIRONMENT CLEAN – AND HOW YOU DO THIS – BENEFITS THE WHOLE COMMUNITY

FEEL-GOOD CLEANING

HOW CLEAN DOES IT NEED TO BE? OPINIONS VARY...

It might be one of the unspoken consequences of the Fall of Man from Paradise: dirt. There is not a hint that Eve cleaned in Paradise. Adam, of course, didn't either. But for whatever reason, dirt is a constant companion of mankind. There isn't much good to say about dirt, except perhaps as the layer of dust on an old wine bottle. And no matter how many times you remove it, dirt keeps coming back.

Perhaps this is one of the reasons why cleaning is often perceived as a negative activity. You clean because you have to. You rarely find pleasure in cleaning and when you do, you probably don't like to admit it. It's not considered particularly cool to be a passionate cleaning devil. Anyone who likes to clean and admits it is considered odd.

Cleaning is one of the last bastions of cultural identity. The way we clean is a clear reflection of cultural diversity. A manufacturer of wipes and scrubbers, who sells his products worldwide, will have looked into this carefully. The expectations of cleaning and wiping cloths vary from country to country. In the global village, everyone sweeps his own doorstep, but each in his own way, determined by tradition and culture.

In Central Europe and North America, the vacuum cleaner, cleaning bucket and mop are the main pillars of domestic cleanliness. But even here, there are differences: while Europeans mainly use a bucket, Americans rinse the mop directly in the sink. All, that is, except Americans with Hispanic roots: they clean like Europeans, with buckets but with lots and lots of water. What both have in common is the use of chemical cleaning agents, often in excessive quantities. What's clean must smell clean. Perhaps that is one of the reasons why allergies are so widespread in these two cleaning cultures and are on the increase.

The market research carried out by our wipes manufacturer will have revealed further insights into cleaning behaviour. In southern European countries, a lot of water and chemicals are generally used for cleaning. Scandinavians, on the other hand, tend to clean dry and attach great importance to the environmental compatibility of their cleaning agents. Belgians and Dutch people click wide fabric cloth-heads onto poles and pull them over tiled floors and laminates – a method that is also favoured in Italy and Spain. The classic mop we are familiar with is almost unknown there.

People build their houses in different ways and with different flooring, according to the climate of the country. High humidity and stone floors require a different cleaning method to low humidity and wooden floors. Some countries with colder climates favour carpets.

The greatest influence on cleaning behaviour, however, is tradition – personified by the mother. The way mother cleans, so the children clean. And because about two-thirds of these cleaning children are female, this tradition is continuously passed on through the generations. With the increasing number of single households, the picture changes only slightly.

Cleaning is something that almost everyone does, only more or less regularly. It is important for well-being, because nobody likes to roll in the dirt. A clean apartment is an apartment in which you feel comfortable, where you literally feel at home.

But when it comes to standards of cleanliness, opinions differ widely. While some are satisfied with superficial cleanliness, maintained by regular vacuuming, floor wiping, toilet cleaning and wiping the shelves in the kitchen, others are constantly on the hunt for dust and streaks. The latter only feel comfortable in a hygienically clean environment. They not only use cloths and cleaning agents, but also disinfectant spray. Thus one could roughly separate the two types: the pragmatic cleaners and the passionate cleaners. Most of us will probably find ourselves somewhere between these two extremes.

However, cleaning can be more than the removal of constantly recurring dirt. Cleaning can help us look closely at our immediate living environment and sharpen our awareness of which things are important to us and which have merely accumulated over time. The important things are the ones treated with care and kept clean and in good condition. You like to clean these things because you like to use them. These are the items that are either regularly or constantly used and are therefore the focus of our attention. A thing that hasn't been cleaned for two years is probably unnecessary, so the frequency of cleaning an object can be an important test when deciding what to keep and what to throw away

This act of cleaning – bringing order into one's own environment – has another dimension. The Japanese, with their Zen Buddhist tradition of concentrating on the essential and consciously performing a particular activity, know 'the way of cleaning' as a spiritual exercise. This spiritual tradition, called 'misogi', sees the main purpose of meditation as cleaning within oneself. It can be seen as a form of psychotherapy by other means. One of the methods is to connect the 'inner cleaning' with the 'outer cleaning', ie. housework. The cleaning thus becomes a kind of active meditation. Concentrating on wiping various surfaces with a damp cloth frees up the mind from compulsive thoughts. The mind becomes an empty – and of course clean – vessel, ready to receive new thoughts in an orderly manner.

Important in this 'misogi' is cleaning with the bare hand and a damp cloth. If you wipe with sufficient pressure, the friction of the damp cloth creates water ions on a solid surface. This is important because life is largely based on water ions. Healthy air contains many water ions. So 'misogi' leads to a healthy environment. It goes without saying that only pure water without industrial detergents is used.

This approach to cleaning is widespread in Japan. Perhaps it also helps that Japanese apartments are very small, and the amount of dirt produced is concentrated in one small room. So you have to clean often to keep the little apartment clean.

This Japanese 'way of cleaning' is one way of looking at the job: as an exercise of mental relaxation. It could start to turn an ordinary, routine or even dreaded task into something that can find the cleaner themself equally improved, through carrying the job out with respect.

Of course cleaning is essential to our well-being and health. And this brings us to the main topic of this book: cleaning agents, detergents that make cleaning easier but do not harm our health. Neither our own health nor that of the environment. Everyone has the right to create grime. But everyone also has a responsibility to remove their grime in a way that does not harm anyone else.

CLEANING CAN DAMAGE YOUR HEALTH

INDUSTRIALLY-PRODUCED CLEANING PRODUCTS OFTEN CONTAIN SUBSTANCES THAT YOU DON'T WANT IN YOUR LIVING ENVIRONMENT.

CLEANING DOES NOT MEAN DISINFECTING

In Western Europe alone, currently around 70,000 products in the field of detergents, cleaning agents and disinfectants are approved for household use.

The average per capita consumption of cleaning products in Germany, for example, is around eleven kilograms per year. Most of it ends up in the sewage, but the rest is distributed around our homes, our clothes and our bodies. That could lead to the conclusion that we are particularly clean. However, because industrially-produced cleaning agents usually contain a whole range of substances that not only guarantee hygienic cleanliness but at the same time have side effects on our health, the question arises: is our dazzlingly clean living environment, which smells of synthetic aromas, really a healthy environment for us? Chemists from environmental and consumer protection organisations regularly examine the cleaning chemicals available on the market. Many products contain combinations of substances for which the term 'poison cocktail' is perhaps not entirely inappropriate.

Especially in those products that smell strongly, toxins lurk. Very few products contain the scent of natural additives such as lemon oil. The vast majority only mimic natural freshness with the help of synthetically assembled molecules, which primarily act on our noses and, even if it is a good product, make only a minor contribution to the cleaning performance of the product. This is one of the differences between natural aromas and synthetic fragrances: the latter only smell strongly at best and at worst cause irritation to the skin, eyes and respiratory tract. But natural aromatics from, for example, essential lemon oil, have immense fat-dissolving power.

It is very difficult for consumers in a supermarket to read from the list of ingredients the proportion of substances that are harmful to health or even toxic. Even if 'bio' is emblazoned on the packaging in giant letters, this is no guarantee of a 'healthy' cleaning agent. In contrast to its use in foodstuffs, the term 'organic' in the case of cleaning agents, is not tied to any particular criteria.

What should a cleaning agent be able to do? It should loosen dirt and make it easy to remove in a solution. What a cleaning agent does not need to do – and in the interests of a healthy living environment should *not* be able to do – is to disinfect your home. The disinfection of a room is necessary in public toilets and clinics, but certainly not in a normal house with residents without infectious diseases. **The fear of bacteria lurking everywhere is not based on scientific knowledge, but on the influence of the advertising of the cleaning agent industry.**

Bacteria are actually everywhere. In our body we carry a considerable amount of them around with us too. Very few of them are harmful to our health, and a functioning immune system can cope with them easily. Many types of bacteria actually promote our health; some are even vital for us. So anyone who treats all bacteria the same and eliminates them chemically, does no good for himself or his health. On the contrary, it appears that children who grow up in a germ-free household suffer much more from a weakened immune system and a whole range of allergies than those whose immune system is allowed to deal with bacteria and germs in a natural way. It is said for good reason that children who grow up with pets are the healthiest children. The immune system of a child who often comes into contact with a dog's tongue is challenged and strengthened. It will be able to cope with other, greater challenges in the future. **There is increasing scientific evidence that children cannot develop their immune system sufficiently in an environment that is too clean.**

The negative effects of a disinfected household are of course not limited to the development of a child's immune system. Many experts believe that household cleaners with antibacterial active ingredients, germicidal additives and integrated disinfectants should not be kept in the cleaning cupboard, but in the poison cabinet. They not only attack the beneficial bacteria on our skin, but also cause harmful bacteria to develop resistance to antibiotics.

As far as disinfectants in household cleaners and their effect on germs are concerned, a recently published study by the University of Massachusetts paints a clear picture: usually only some of the germs are killed by the disinfectant cleaner. The surviving germs are then able to adapt, to develop resistance. This means that these germs will in future become immune to this disinfectant cleaning agent, so its use will be completely pointless.

TERPENES AND ETHYLENE GLYCOL

If a room smells of cleaning agents, it is usually assumed that the room is clean. If the room is not sufficiently ventilated, it can still smell for days after cleaning.

That clean, hygienic smell from chemical cleaning products actually means something completely different: that the room is saturated with chemicals! Even bio-cleaners have their risks. Some detergents that 'naturally' smell like oranges or lemons get this scent from the terpenes they contain. Those cleaning agents that leave a breath of fresh forest air in the room fall into this category. Their scent comes from pine resins. Resins and terpenes are generally not considered toxic. However, they have a high allergenic potential and they react chemically with ozone. Ozone is constantly present in the air, in increased concentrations on hot summer days and in rooms where copiers, printers or electric air fresheners are used. The biochemical reaction of terpenes and resins in contact with ozone leads to a number of toxic compounds such as formaldehyde, which is believed to cause cancer. In addition, toxic fine dust is also produced, the concentration of which depends on the respective ozone value.

Today, it is accepted that conventional cleaning agents contain unhealthy or even dangerous substances. The most common are various glycol ethers. These are alcoholic compounds with high fat-dissolving and disinfection powers. They smell pleasantly fresh or are odourless. However, the most widely-used ethylene glycol has the unwelcome property that our body absorbs it through the skin and through respiration. The consequences range from irritation of the eyes, mucous membranes and respiratory tract to dizziness and persistent unnatural fatigue. If ethylene glycol is used for a long period of time, permanent damage to blood cells, bone marrow and the reproductive system may occur. Ethylene glycol can be a particularly dangerous ingredient in conventional cleaning agents because it is odourless, so not noticed.

INVISIBLE AND ODOURLESS: NANOPARTICLES

The use of nanoparticles in detergents is still relatively new and their health effects have only been researched to a limited extent.

Nanoparticles are particles with a diameter of less than a millionth of a millimetre, and they work primarily because of their tiny size.

If a material is shredded into ever smaller particles, its surface area increases. A powder of nanoparticles therefore has a huge surface. It offers its surroundings far more surface contact and this makes it more effective. This is also due to the fact that the molecules on the surface of a particle have different physical properties to those inside the particle. The surface molecules are not completely surrounded by neighbouring molecules of the same type, but they 'rub shoulders with' the molecules of the substance surrounding them. It is these surface molecules that determine the properties of a nanoparticle. Because of the unimaginably tiny size of a nanoparticle, there are considerably more surface molecules than there are those inside the particle. Nanoparticles of zinc oxide, for example, absorb UV radiation, but larger particles of the same substance do not.

Cleaning agents mainly contain nanoparticles of silver. They have the ability to kill bacteria and germs and are therefore used in hygiene cleaning products for kitchen, bathroom and toilet. At first glance, the advantages of nanoparticles made of silver seem immense: no harmful disinfectants, no chemical contamination of the room air and the fact that it is considered unlikely bacteria and germs can form any resistance to the effects of nanosilver.

Nanoparticles are just as convincing in floor cleaning agents, especially for laminate and parquet floors. As soon as the cleaning agent hits the floor, nanoparticles settle into even the tiniest joints and cracks and do not let a drop of water come into contact with the sensitive wood. Swelling parquet floors are thus a thing of the past. Or, to take another example: a glass cleaner for streak-free shiny windows and mirrors, which puts a protective film of nanoparticles over the glass pane and thus reduces future dirt.

The chemical industry is continually developing new products for household cleaning that are pepped up with nanoparticles. You usually won't find them in the list of ingredients. But for some manufacturers, the great effectiveness of nanoparticles is used as a convincing sales argument.

Scientists warn against particles that are a thousand times smaller than fine dust. There is still a lot of research to be done before anyone can say with certainty whether or not the tiny particles penetrate the human body through inhalation, through the skin or through residues on crockery and cutlery and what damage they can do there.

First results from recent experiments should, however, sound alarm bells. For example, it is already considered certain that our body's defence system does not recognise penetrating nanoparticles because it is aimed at protecting against larger foreign bodies. Nanoparticles of this kind do not occur in nature, so no natural defence strategy has been developed by the body.

Inhaled nanoparticles can get into the smallest alveoli. Normally foreign bodies are enveloped and rendered harmless by the special defence cells called macrophages. Nanoparticles, on the other hand, are too small to be recognised by macrophages.

The lung is not the only organ endangered by nanoparticles because, via the lungs, nanoparticles could pass with ease into the bloodstream. Only a wall a thousandth of a millimetre thick separates the vesicles from the blood vessels. Nanoparticles have no problem penetrating this wall. The amount of nanoparticles that enter the blood depends on the material, size and surface properties of the particles. Nanoparticles can also penetrate the blood through the intestinal wall. Healthy skin, on the other hand, is considered impermeable to nanoparticles.

Science is only gradually discovering what nanoparticles can do once we have them in our blood stream. A team led by Professor Anna von Mikecz at the Institute for Environmental Medicine Research at the University of Düsseldorf was able to prove that certain types of nanoparticles in sufficiently high concentrations interfere with the functions of the cell nucleus (press release of the Leibniz Institute for Environmental Medicine Research January 2014). Other possible effects are circulatory damage and even brain damage. The experts are unanimous in their view that nanoparticles in household cleaners harbour a risk potential whose full extent cannot yet be assessed.

Other additives in conventional cleaning agents that have recently made a name for themselves are microplastics. Microscopically small plastic beads are used to increase friction during scrubbing – in toothpastes as well as in scouring cream and toilet cleaners. After it has fulfilled its task, this microplastic is mostly discharged into the wastewater. However, most water treatment plants are not able to eliminate microplastics from the wastewater so it can enter rivers unhindered. Fish and sea creatures with plastic balls in their organs are one of the consequences.

Since this problem was first recognised, measures have been taken to tackle it and, given the damage already caused by microplastics, its use is already being limited. The future will show whether this restriction is fully enforced.

HOMEMADE HOUSEHOLD CLEANERS: A BIT OF BACKGROUND SCIENCE

THOSE WHO DO NOT WANT TO DAMAGE THEIR HEALTH AND POLLUTE THE ENVIRONMENT HAVE AN ALTERNATIVE TO INDUSTRIALLY-PRODUCED CLEANING AGENTS. MAKE YOUR OWN.

Industrially-produced household cleaners have been around for only about a century. In 1884 the world's first packaged, branded household soap was created at the Sunlight soap factory in northern England. Meanwhile, the first synthetic detergent was introduced in 1930, dishwashing detergents were launched in 1948, and the first synthetic detergent to do entirely without soap was only introduced in 1952. So the history of industrial detergent chemistry is relatively young.

Before the chemical industry started to produce all kinds of household cleaning agents, these products were made either in small factories and were mostly soap-based, or they were made in the household itself. These cleaning agents had one obvious advantage: they did not harm the health of the residents or the environment.

In order to follow this tradition of 'healthy cleaning', we first need a little bit of chemistry, because the dissolving of dirt is a chemical process.

The simplest and most environmentally-friendly cleaning agent is pure water. Water has the ability to dissolve and absorb substances. But only water-soluble substances. Many substances are only fat-soluble, and some are only alcohol-soluble. So if the dirt consists entirely or partially of greasy components, pure water has no effect. Pure water is pH-neutral, ie. neither acidic nor alkaline. The rule of thumb is:

'Like dissolves like', which means that fatty components can only be removed with fat-soluble agents, such as soaps produced from fats.

THE pH

The pH value is critical when it comes to cleaning. It indicates the proportion of oxygen ions in a solution. The further the pH value deviates from the neutral value pH 7, the more reactive a solution is.

The pH Scale

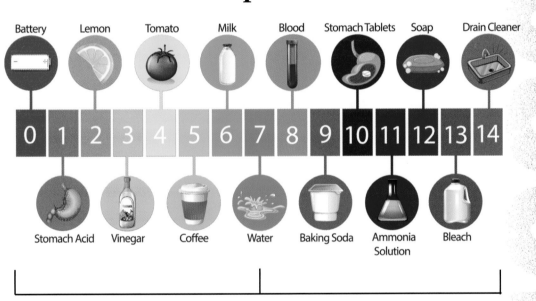

The range from pH1 to pH7
are the **acids**

The range from pH7 to pH14
are the **alkalis**

Acids contain positively charged hydrogen particles which attract where they find negatively charged particles, to balance their charge. Alkalis have an excess of negatively-charged particles which are attracted to positively charged particles in their environment.

The following examples are intended to illustrate the scale of pH values:

Our stomachs are very acidic with a pH of 1, lemon juice has a pH of 2, vinegar has a pH of 3, wine has an average pH of 4, coffee has a pH of 5 and mineral water has a pH of 6. The surface of our skin usually has a pH of 5.5. Only distilled water reaches a neutral pH of 7. The alkalis begin above pH 7. From slightly alkaline solutions such as our blood with an average pH of 7.4, seawater with a pH of 8, soap with a pH of about 10 to strongly alkaline caustic soda with a pH of 14.

Because the pH scale is logarithmic, mineral water with a pH of 6 is ten times more acidic than distilled water with a neutral pH of 7, for example. Coffee with a pH of 5 is a hundred times more acidic than distilled water.

In order to use the right detergent, you must first be aware of the type of dirt you want to remove. Greasy dirt requires a high pH value, such as soap, soap solutions or washing soda. Cleaning agents based on soap or soda are therefore the ideal fat solvents. They are suitable for all areas of the household that are mainly soiled with grease: cookers, ovens, sinks and dishes, kitchen floors and the edges of bathtubs.

A low pH value such as vinegar has no effect on greasy dirt. Therefore cleaning agents based on acetic acid (vinegar essence) are particularly suitable for removing calciferous staining, such as the tarred stains in cups and jugs, limescale deposits in washbasins and taps, but also as water softeners for dishwashing and washing laundry. Detergents based on vinegar or acetic acid are effective against mould growth and are a mild disinfectant that eliminates bacteria, germs and spores.

Because both very low and very high pH values can cause burns to the skin, it is very important to always wear gloves when cleaning – whether you are working with acidic vinegar-based detergents or alkaline soap-based detergents. The fact that a cleaning agent is of natural origin and does not harm health or the environment in its side effects does not mean that handling it is completely safe.

SAPONINS VERSUS SURFACTANTS

Before the industry produced household cleaners in large quantities, liquid soaps were made either from saponins – foam-making substances such as those found in soapwort – or from soft soap boiled from fats in small factories. In any case, saponins were the detergents which de-greased.

Today you can find in every supermarket liquid cleaners and even hand soaps which do not contain saponins and often even advertise themselves as 'soap-free'. This has created a bad reputation for soap. Soap has a high pH value of about 10 and is therefore suspected of attacking the protective acid coating of the skin. However, the desired de-greasing effect – in other words, the cleaning effect of the soap – depends on this high pH value. A soap with a lower pH value would be pointless. For hand soaps, the answer lies in additional grease. So as well as saponified fat, these nourishing soaps also contain a certain amount of unsaponified fats which protect the natural oil coating on the skin or at least help the skin to restore it.

Soap-free cleaning agents use active washing substances with a neutral to slightly acid pH value. These detergents work by reducing the surface tension and thus act as a 'bridge' between dirt and the washing solution. These washing substances belong to the group called surfactants. Soaps are also surfactants, but the term surfactant covers a much larger group than just the soaps. Surfactants frequently include quaternary ammonium compounds. The disadvantage of these cationic surfactants is that they are 'biocidal' (Greek for 'life killing') and can cause resistance to pathogens as well as allergies.

Soaps, on the other hand, are among the anionic surfactants. A soap molecule consists of a water-repellent and a water-attracting part. With water, soap forms so-called micelles. These ensure that an emulsion is formed from water and fat droplets. This mixture of fat and water can then simply be rinsed away.

In very hard water, however, the micelles have a problem: their polar ends can be blocked by calcium and magnesium ions, forming water-insoluble scum. However, the lime content of our normal drinking water is rarely sufficient for this. So you only need to use a water softener for very hard water. From an ecological point of view, the tendency to form scum has an advantage. Scum and fatty acids are not only insoluble, they are also not surface-active, so that they can be easily decomposed by micro-organisms.

All these various risks and undesirable side effects can be avoided in homemade detergents. Doing it yourself not only brings healthy cleanliness into our living environment, it also saves money. The raw materials for homemade household cleaners are very cheap to buy. But there's nothing cheap about what you can make from them. Quite the opposite: they are high-quality products which you rarely get to buy!

RAW MATERIALS AND UTENSILS

The things you need to make your own cleaning agents are usually already in your kitchen.

If you want to make your own household cleaners, you don't need a chemical laboratory or a huge stock of raw materials. You can get by with just a few basic materials, which are combined in different ways, depending on the intended use.

VINEGAR

VINEGAR FORMS A GOOD BASIS FOR ALL CLEANING PURPOSES
EXCEPT TO REMOVE GREASE.

Vinegar is generally produced by the fermentation of alcoholic liquids using special bacteria. Wine and fruit vinegar produced by alcoholic fermentation contains about 5 per cent acetic acid. Vinegar essence – usually 25 per cent – has a significantly higher acid content. It is produced artificially and may only be used in appropriate dilutions for food. But as a base for cleaning agents, vinegar essence has the advantage that, depending on the degree of contamination, the degree of acidity can be adjusted by dilution. For cleaning purposes, vinegar essence should only be used undiluted if very strong calcifications have to be removed. The evaporation of the undiluted vinegar essence can irritate the respiratory tract and mucous membranes, so should only be used in well-ventilated rooms.

In most cleaning products, a vinegar essence is diluted one to four with water. Alternatively, even a cheap white spirit or fruit vinegar is sufficient.

Vinegar is above all a good glass cleaner. Heavily soiled window panes can be cleaned with water and a strong dash of vinegar – it's streak free and effortless. Our grandmothers used crumpled newspaper to finish the drying job, streak fee. It still can't be beaten for that purpose today.

Vinegar itself does not dissolve fat, but in combination with hot water it is a healthy dishwashing detergent because it is residue free. The aggressive cleaners from the supermarket are not only unfriendly to our hands, they can also leave traces of surfactants on the dishes. Particularly questionable in this respect are the so-called 'rinse aids'. They coat dishes with a film that reduces the surface tension of water and thus ensures that the drops of water roll off the dishes better.

Due to its disinfectant properties, vinegar can be used as a base for toilet cleaners. Vinegar can also be useful for laundry: as a fabric softener it not only makes the laundry soft and fragrant, but also freshens up the colours by removing any limescale residues.

What certainly doesn't go together is vinegar and soap. Online you can find recipes that want to mix these opposite poles of cleaning chemistry into one product. That's nonsense! If soap and vinegar are mixed together, the result is a greyish, cloudy broth with greasy, light lumps. I m sure you wouldn't want to clean anything with that!

SOAPS AND SOAP FLAKES

SOAP-BASED DETERGENTS ARE THE FIRST CHOICE AGAINST ANY TYPE OF GREASE OR GREASY DIRT.

The base soap can come in various forms for our homemade cleaning agents: as liquid soap, as pure curd soap or as soap flakes. You can produce liquid soap

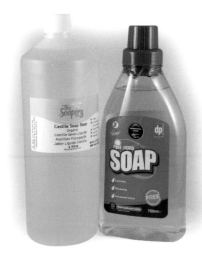

yourself without much effort, from any fat or oil mixed with caustic soda. But we will come to this in a later chapter.

The cheapest and simplest soap base to make is a block of curd soap. The purity is important, so no fragrances should be added to curd soap. For use in liquid detergents, the solid block of soap is simply grated into flakes. If this is too much work for you, you can buy ready-grated soap flakes and process them according to the recipe. **The important thing about soap flakes is that they must consist of pure curd soap.** You can get curd soap in handicraft shops, online, in health food shops and chemists.

A variant of the curd soap is Castile soap. This is a purely vegetable product made from coconut or olive oil. Castile soap is available in organic shops and good pharmacies or online, both as liquid soap and in solid form.

WASHING SODA (SODIUM CARBONATE, SODA CRYSTALS OR SODA ASH)

... IS A TRADITIONAL PRODUCT FOR CLEANING LAUNDRY.

You can get it in organic hardware stores, pharmacies or health food stores, and more recently, in a few supermarkets. Its chemical name is sodium carbonate. It dissolves stains and grease, softens the laundry and is also effective in other applications such as floor cleaners.

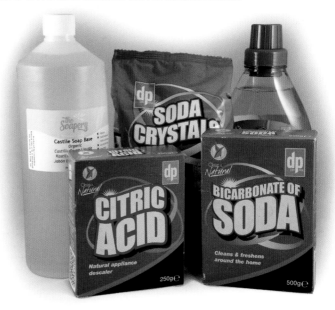

BICARBONATE OF SODA (BAKING SODA – NB NOT BAKING POWDER)

SODIUM BICARBONATE IS THE CHEMICAL NAME FOR BAKING SODA, AS IT IS NOT ONLY NEEDED FOR CERTAIN HOMEMADE DETERGENTS, BUT ALSO, IN THE KITCHEN, FOR BAKING.

You can find it in almost every supermarket or grocery store among the baking ingredients where it will cost more than in a hardware shop. Do not confuse it with baking *powder* which contains mainly sodium bicarbonate, but also other ingredients. If *sodium bicarbonate* is mentioned in the recipes, only *pure* bicarbonate of soda should be used, not baking powder. Bicarbonate of soda is also much cheaper than baking powder, which is sold in much smaller quantities.

GLYCERINE

... is an alcoholic compound obtained by separating fats into fatty acids and glycerol. It is used in some detergent recipes and is available from pharmacies, online and in DIY stores.

TURPENTINE

... is obtained by distilling the thick resin of various conifers, and it is used as a solvent.

BEESWAX

... is a nourishing and pleasantly fragrant additive for wood care products and floor polish.

It is available in the form of small blocks in health food shops, also from craft shops and online. Beeswax has a practically unlimited shelf life, so you can stock up on it freely.

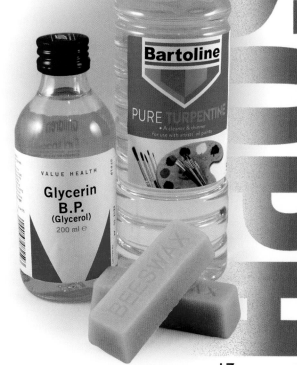

HERBS

Among the multitude of herbs that thrive in the wild, in the garden and in pots on balconies and terraces, there are a number of herbs that are invaluable in detergents.

Rosemary, sage, lavender, mint or lemon balm are among these. Their dried leaves and flowers can be used to make fragrant scouring powder, effective carpet cleaning powder, air fresheners and as a fragrant yet antibacterial and germ-killing ingredient to a range of household cleaners, from all-purpose cleaners to scouring agents for the bathroom. All herbs containing essential oils are suitable. If you can't use your own herbs, you can buy dried ones at little cost.

HOW TO MAKE A DECOCTION

Whenever oil extracts or decoctions of herbs are mentioned in recipes, they have always been made from dried herbs. Fresh herbs contain water, which isn't good for our purposes. Firstly, the water content cannot be precisely estimated because it depends on many factors – including the phase and position of the moon at the time of harvest. Secondly, the water content carries the risk of mould formation.

A decoction of herbs will extract the essential oils and other ingredients from the stems, larger leaves or crushed, dried root parts.

To make a decoction, tip the dried plant material into a stainless steel or enamel pan (not aluminium!), pour water over it to about three times the volume of the plant material, place the pan on the hob and heat until it boils. Then turn the heat down to a gentle simmer with the lid on for about 15 to 20 minutes. Remove from heat and let the decoction cool a little before straining it into a suitable vessel. You can use the decoction as soon as it has cooled down to room temperature, but you can also store it in a well-sealed container for up to three weeks in the fridge for later use.

In a variety of recipes, an infusion of herbs can be used instead of plain water. In principle, it is nothing more than a very strong herbal tea. Tender plant parts such as flowers and young leaves can also be used. Pour boiling water over them and let them steep for about 15 minutes. A heaped tablespoon of dried herbs to a cup of water is about the right ratio.

ESSENTIAL OILS

The essential oils of the herbs contain active ingredients in the highest concentration.

Many herbs have antibiotic, antiviral and antiseptic properties or work against fungi and fungal spores. If you want to transfer these properties to a detergent in a more concentrated form, you can use the pure essential oils of the herbs.

Essential oils are not only effective in terms of hygiene when it comes to a cleaning agent, they actually make a contribution to its cleaning performance. Essential citrus oil, for example, has immense fat-dissolving power, because it is an *oil*. Essential oils also give a cleaning agent its individual scent, which fills the room

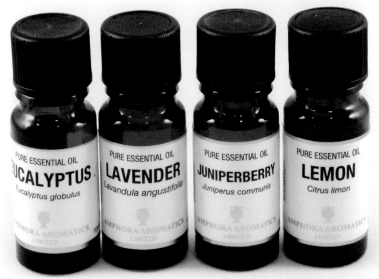

during the cleaning process, so you can add your favourite fragrance to the living area, kitchen, bathroom and toilet. It is important to use only genuine, pure and undiluted essential oils. Synthetically-produced scented oils might smell lovely, but they have no other effect.

Essential oils are relatively expensive but, due to their very high concentration, only a few drops at a time are used.

Essential oils are complex substances which only unlock their full effect when they interact. It has not yet been possible to produce essential oils in the laboratory with anything near the same effectiveness.

The most important of these essential oil ingredients are:

TERPENES

They have an antiseptic and anti-inflammatory effect. They are found in particularly high concentrations in lavender, coriander, peppermint, thyme and eucalyptus – to name just a few.

PHENOLS

Phenols kill bacteria and germs. They are particularly concentrated in clove, cinnamon and thyme, for example.

Certain essential oils also contain ketones (the essential oils of rosemary, peppermint or caraway), aldehydes (lemon grass, lemon, orange) as well as alcohols, esters (an acid compound) and cineole (eucalyptol), often in a variety of different compounds.

The most effective essential oils for household cleaning are thyme oil, oregano oil, eucalyptus oil, lavender oil, citrus oil, sandalwood oil and tea tree oil. They are not only antibacterial and germicidal, but they also have properties that increase the cleaning performance of our homemade household cleaners. Because essential oils also work through their fragrance and because that is very subjective, the key essential oils are listed here according to their hygienic function. This allows you to choose your preferred essential oils based on both their effects and their fragrance.

ANTIBACTERIAL ESSENTIAL OILS

Camomile, Camphor, Cardamom, Cinnamon, Citronella, Clove, Eucalyptus, Ginger, Hyssop, Juniper, Lavender, Lemon, Lemon Grass, Lime, Marjoram, Orange, Oregano, Peppermint, Pine, Rosemary, Sage, Sandalwood, Savory, Tea Tree, Thyme, Verbena.

FUNGICIDAL ESSENTIAL OILS

Eucalyptus, Hyssop, Juniper, Lavender, Lemon, Myrtle, Oregano, Sage, Sandalwood, Savory, Tea Tree, Thyme.

ANTIVIRAL ESSENTIAL OILS

Balm, Cinnamon, Clove, Cypress, Eucalyptus, Hyssop, Lavender, Lemon, Oregano, Patchouli, Sandalwood, Tea Tree, Thyme.

Basic materials for the production of essential oils are pure, natural products, which can vary according to their growing conditions. As a result, there are certain *quality* differences between pure essential oils, but these are not so important when it comes to cleaning agents. They mainly affect the quality of the fragrance, which is important for aromatherapy, for example, but not for household cleaners.

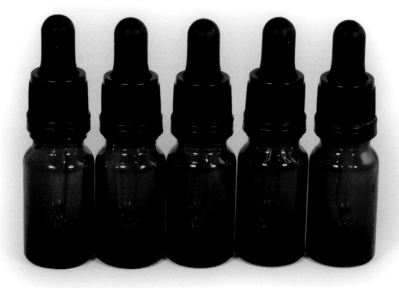

It is important to buy only pure, undiluted essential oils. They should not be mixed with a carrier oil – usually almond or jojoba oil. Essential oils are sold in coloured, mostly brown glass bottles because they must be protected from the effects of light. If they are stored in a cool and dark place, the effectiveness of some essential oils is almost unlimited. Citrus oils, however, can only be kept for about one year. The oils usually come in dropper bottles, the lid of which already contains a pipette, which is helpful when measuring the amount of drops that are specified in the recipe for your homemade detergent. Because essential oils are highly concentrated, it is important to follow this quantity exactly. If you use more than the amount indicated, you do not increase the effectiveness. On the contrary, too high a concentration can lead to skin irritations and irritations of the respiratory tract as a side effect.

Essential oils contain the active ingredients of the respective plants in the highest concentration. To give an example: a single drop of essential camomile oil contains the active ingredients for about 30 cups of camomile tea! Essential oils should only be used diluted appropriately to their use. Dealing with them requires a certain degree of care. They should be stored like medicines: out of reach for children and pets. Certain essential oils can also trigger allergies in predisposed people. A good test of this is to apply a tiny amount of the essential oil in the crook of the arm and to watch for any reaction to the skin. For small children and during pregnancy, the use of essential oils should generally be avoided. In many recipes, essential oils can be omitted without affecting the effectiveness too much.

Further ingredients listed in certain recipes, such as citric acid or tartaric acid, are available in groceries, supermarkets and online.

USEFUL EQUIPMENT

You will find most of the equipment you need to make your own household cleaners in your kitchen. So you will only need to purchase one or two items for this purpose. And if you do, you can certainly use them for other kitchen and household jobs.

KITCHEN SCALES

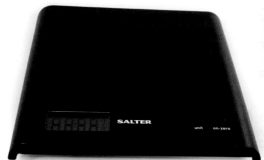

Indispensable for precise weighing of ingredients. A measuring range up to three or five kilograms is useful, but more important is the accuracy of one gram in the lower measuring range, up to about 200 grams. Especially if you are thinking of making your own soap and liquid soap – this accuracy is essential. Normal digital kitchen scales are inexpensive and meet these requirements.

MEASURING JUG

When adding water or other liquids, the quantity should not be estimated, but measured as accurately as possible. Measuring cups or measuring glasses are the suitable equipment for this purpose. Whether they are made of glass or plastic doesn't matter, because today it can be assumed that those made of plastic are also largely resistant to acids and alkalis.

MIXER, BLENDER OR HAND BLENDER

Pretty much everything we do ourselves in terms of cleaning agents requires intensive mixing of the ingredients. If you don't want to do this in a long, tiring process with a hand whisk, use a mixer. A hand blender or a stick blender is ideal. With an electric whisk you should remove one of the two whisks. But no matter what kind of mixer you use, the right speed is the lowest speed!

ATOMISER, SPRAY BOTTLE

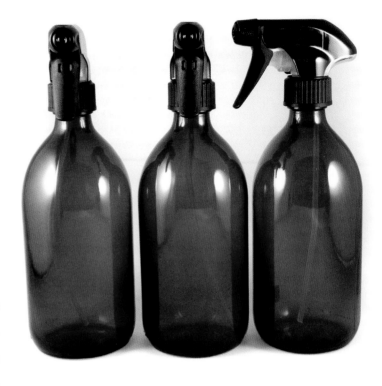

Many of our self-made cleaning agents are sprayed in liquid form onto the surface to be cleaned. This is the best way to avoid over-dosing. Suitable spray pump bottles can be bought cheaply in DIY stores, hardware shops and, of course, online. Because they are usually available in different colours, each detergent can be assigned its own bottle. Nevertheless, you should also label them.

BOWLS, PANS

... in different sizes are necessary for the production of different recipes. They should be made of glass or stainless steel. Plastic or aluminium bowls are not suitable for this purpose. With plastic bowls, you cannot be sure that they are insensitive to acids and alkalis, and aluminium can react chemically with our detergent ingredients.

CONTAINERS FOR DETERGENTS

Bottles and jars with screw caps or clip caps are the ideal containers for your homemade household cleaners. However, you can also reuse suitable empty containers of conventional cleaning agents. If you go down this route, they must be well washed and dried so that residues of industrially-produced cleaners cannot contaminate your homemade ones.

For vinegar-based cleaning agents, containers with metal lids should not be used as this can cause oxidisation due to the evaporating acetic acid. Plastic containers are more suitable for cleaning agents containing vinegar.

In all events, careful and accurate labelling of the containers is recommended. There should be no possibility of confusion. It is best to stick a label with the name and ingredients of the cleaning agent on its container. You can use normal stickers from the stationery trade. Because these are usually not waterproof, they should be covered with transparent adhesive tape.

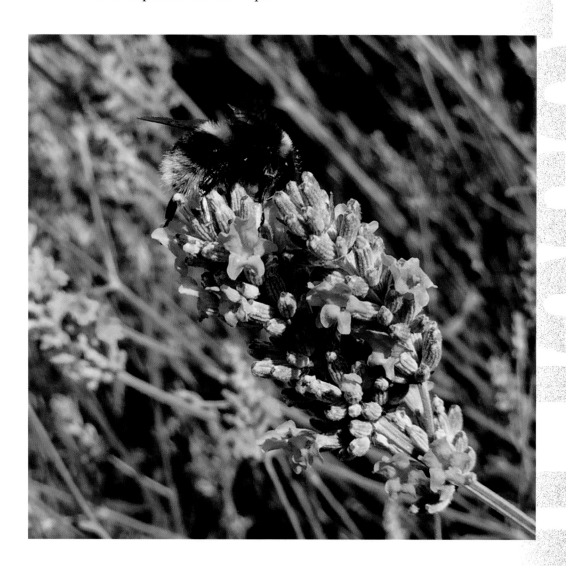

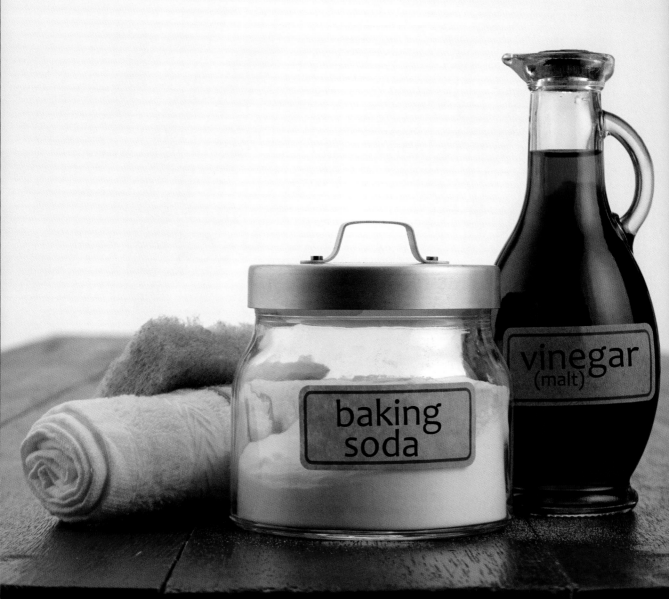

CHAPTER TWO

MULTI-PURPOSE CLEANERS

You'll need this multi-purpose cleaning hero again and again

LIQUID ALL-PURPOSE CLEANER

Something sticky here, a few splashes of grease there, the work surface in the kitchen, the washbasin in the bathroom, lino or tiled floors, a windowsill – everything that is quickly wiped clean calls for the all-purpose cleaner. The term 'multi-purpose cleaner' is more correct, because of course it is not suitable for *all* purposes. It doesn't need to be, because we can use special cleaning agents for special cleaning tasks.

It is ideal if the multi-purpose cleaner is of such a thin consistency that it can also be filled into a spray bottle. Then you can simply spray it onto the surface to be cleaned, wipe it with a cloth and you're done. This type of application is the most economical as you're not tempted to use more cleaner than you need.

LIQUID MULTI-PURPOSE CLEANER WITH LEMON

10g washing soda
1 litre water
juice of a lemon and/or
10 drops essential citrus oil

This cleaner leaves behind not only cleanliness, but also a light lemon scent.

Pour a litre of water over the washing soda in a large bowl and completely dissolve by stirring it thoroughly with a whisk. The squeezed juice of a lemon should be poured through a coffee filter to remove even the finest particles of flesh. Then add it to the soda solution and stir again vigorously. Freshly squeezed lemon juice has a shorter shelf life, so if you are using that, don't make too much at a time: but it will last several weeks. As an alternative to lemon juice, you can use ten drops of essential citrus oil. Either way, you get a concentrated cleaner, which you fill into a storage jar or bottle and keep cool. For use, the cleaner concentrate is diluted with three to four parts of water and filled into a spray bottle.

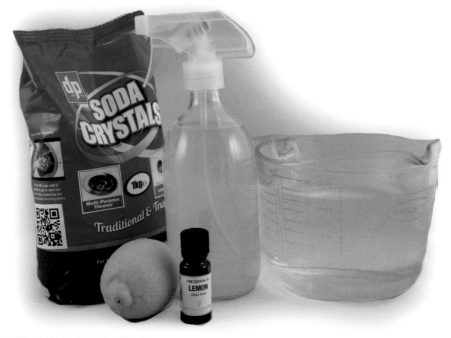

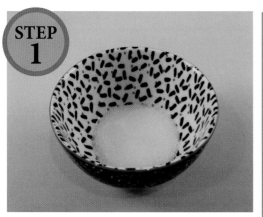

STEP 1

Weigh soda

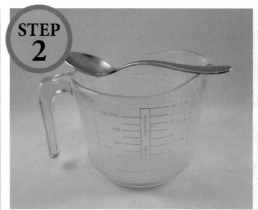

STEP 2

Pour over the water

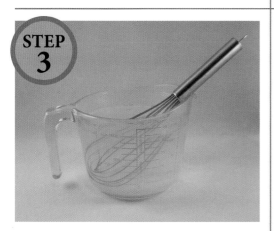

STEP 3

Stir well

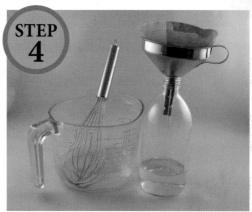

STEP 4

Pour lemon juice through coffee filter

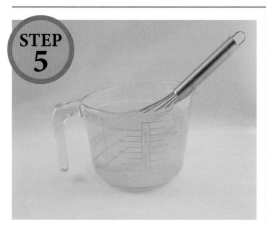

STEP 5

Add lemon juice to the soda solution.
Stir well again...

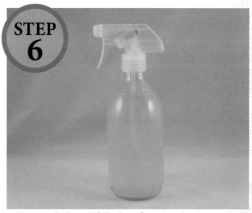

STEP 6

... and then fill the finished cleaner
into a spray bottle.

LIQUID MULTI-PURPOSE VINEGAR-BASED CLEANER ////////////

200ml white vinegar
300ml water
10 drops essential citrus oil

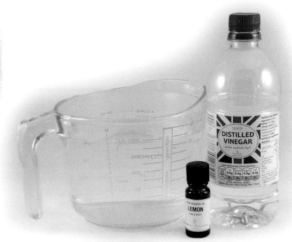

Quickly produced and effective: stir vinegar and water together, add essential citrus oil, stir again, fill into the spray bottle – done!

CLEANING CONCENTRATE WITH VINEGAR ESSENCE ////////////

250ml vinegar essence
  (any white vinegar with 20-25 % acetic acid)
250ml water
15 drops essential tea tree or thyme oil

All ingredients are mixed together, stirred well and the concentrated cleaner is filled into a storage bottle. For use, it is diluted with one to three parts of water, depending on the intended use.

This cleaner can also cope with limescale deposits on taps and sinks and has a highly disinfecting effect.

SOAP-BASED MULTI-PURPOSE CLEANERS

MULTI-PURPOSE CLEANER WITH CURD SOAP

Soap-based all-purpose cleaners are more viscous and therefore not suitable in spray bottles. It is best to fill them into a bottle with a screw cap or swing stopper. This cleaner is either applied in small quantities directly to the cloth or dotted sparingly over the surface to be cleaned. A soap-based cleaner always requires wiping with clear water to remove fine soap residues. See page 32 for this recipe.

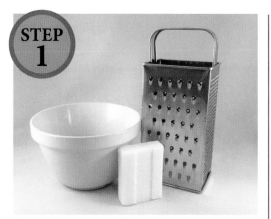

STEP 1

Grate the block of curd soap into flakes. Alternatively you can use soap flakes.

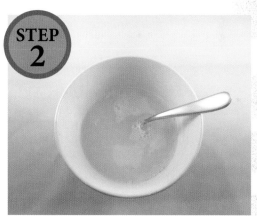

STEP 2

Pour boiling water over it.

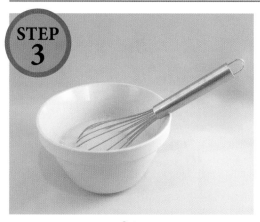

STEP 3

Stir

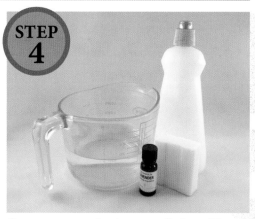

STEP 4

Stir in essential oil, stir well, then fill into suitable bottles.

MULTI-PURPOSE CLEANER WITH CURD SOAP

30g grated curd soap or soap flakes
1 litre water
10 drops essential lavender oil

A piece of curd soap is grated into fine flakes, boiling water is poured over it in a large heatproof bowl and and stirred until the soap has completely dissolved. After the soap solution has cooled down, add essential citrus or lavender oil, depending on your personal taste. You now have a cleaner concentrate that thickens after a few hours to a gel-like consistency. For use it can be diluted with up to five parts water.

POWER CLEANER WITH SOAP AND SODA

40g grated curd soap or soap flakes
10g washing soda
1 water (2 x 0.5 litres)
10 drops essential citrus oil

Two pans or large glass bowls are needed to produce this power cleaner concentrate: in one pot, the soap flakes are covered with half a litre of boiling water and completely dissolved by stirring with the whisk. In the other bowl or pan, pour half a litre of cold water over the soda powder and dissolve it

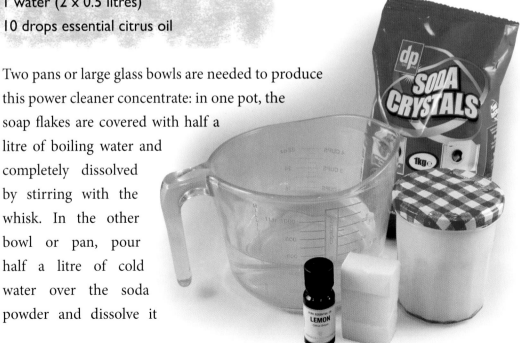

completely by stirring. As soon as the soap solution has cooled down a little, pour the two solutions together and stir well. After cooling to room temperature, stir in the essential citrus oil and you have a cleaning concentrate that can be diluted with three parts water to use even with stubborn greasy dirt.

WET WIPES

THE CONVENIENT CLEANER

Wet wipe cloths are a very practical thing when a surface needs to be wiped quickly to make it clean and germ-free. You don't have to buy expensive wet wipes – and at the same time use a largely unknown chemical cocktail – you can make them yourself simply and cheaply while still maintaining a healthy living environment by using harmless ingredients.

Cellulose cloths are available in jumbo rolls, but many disposable towels are made of pure cellulose and are therefore ideally suited. You simply cut the wipes to the desired size and soak them with a homemade detergent. These wet wipes should be stored in such a way that they do not dry out and that the cleaning agent does not evaporate wastefully into the environment. Their storage container needs to be airtight – you could re-use an existing plastic wipes container. Ideal are biscuit tins – in which the moist cloths can be folded and stacked on top of each other. The wet wipes can also be stored folded in plastic zip bags, available in every supermarket. Like tin boxes, they can be reused over a long period of time.

WIPES WITH ROSEMARY SCENT

100ml white vinegar
100ml water
10 drops essential rosemary oil
20 cellulose wipes (about 30 x 30 cm)

All liquid ingredients are mixed in a bowl. Then stack a suitable number of cut cloths on top of each other and place them in the bowl. It takes some time until all the cloths are soaked with the liquid. Place the damp cloths immediately into their container – biscuit tin or zip bag – and pour over any remaining liquid. Keep in a carefully closed container until use.

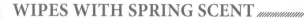

WIPES WITH SPRING SCENT

100ml red clover decoction
100ml white vinegar
10 drops of essential oil (thyme, sage, balm)
20 cellulose wipes (about 30 x 30 cm)

Take a heaped tablespoon of dried red clover, place in a large glass bowl and pour over 100ml boiling water. Allow to infuse for about twelve minutes, strain, cool briefly then mix with the vinegar and the essential oil. The cut cloths are soaked in the liquid, as described above, and put in their container. Pour any of the remaining liquid over the cloths in the container so they remain moist.

TRAVEL WIPES

Travel wipes are invaluable whether in the car or for the restaurant toilet seat. For such purposes, here are suitable travel wipes with antibacterial properties.

200ml camomile decoction
5g bicarbonate of soda
15 drops essential camomile oil
20 cellulose wipes (about 30 x 30cm)

To make the decoction, pour just over 200ml boiling water onto two tablespoons of dried camomile flowers, leave to soak for about ten to twelve

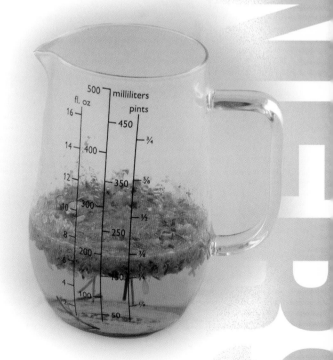

minutes, strain and allow to cool. Then dissolve the soda in the camomile decoction by stirring well and add the essential camomile oil. In a bowl, stack cellulose cloths cut to size on top of each other and pour the liquid over them. As soon as the cloths have absorbed the liquid thoroughly, you can pack them in small zip bags.

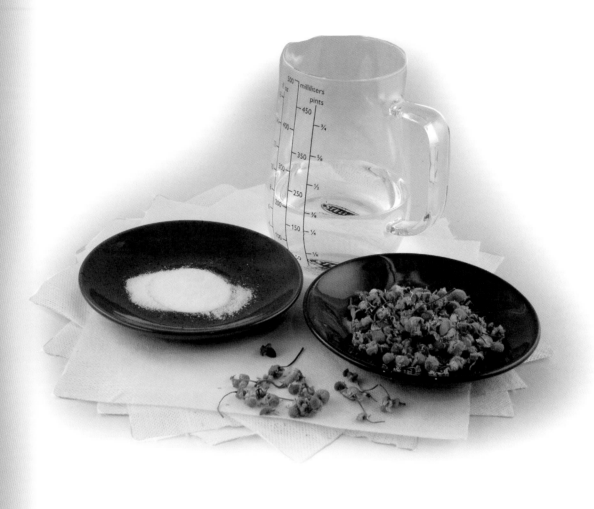

OIL WIPES FOR GREASY THINGS

Anyone who repairs things frequently will not be able to avoid oil or grease on their hands and work surfaces. For greasy dirt you need wiping cloths with a grease-dissolving cleaning agent, ie. oil cloths.

150ml rapeseed, sunflower or olive oil
10 drops essential citrus oil
20 cellulose wipes (about 30 x 30cm)

Mix the essential oil thoroughly with the other oil and pour over the cloths that have been stacked in a bowl and cut to size. Soak only a few cloths at a time and leave them in the oil for a long time. They can be stored in plastic bags until needed.

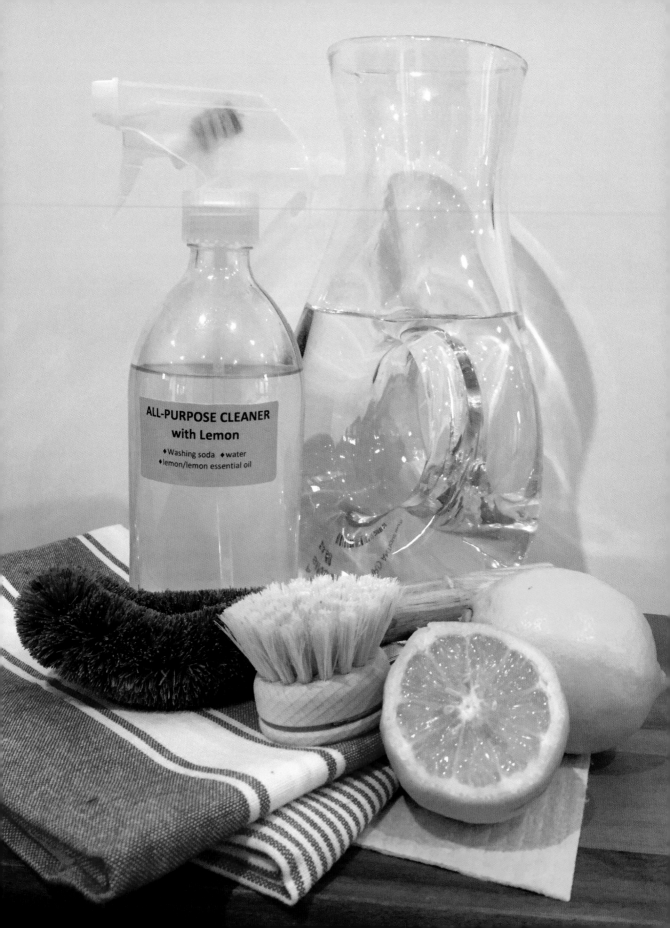

ALL-PURPOSE CLEANER
with Lemon

◆Washing soda ◆water
◆lemon/lemon essential oil

CHAPTER THREE

THE KITCHEN

IN THE KITCHEN, SPECIAL EMPHASIS IS PLACED ON CLEANLINESS. THIS DOES NOT MEAN, HOWEVER, THAT YOU ARE DEPENDENT ON INDUSTRIALLY-PRODUCED CLEANERS AND DETERGENTS

THE KITCHEN

The kitchen is more than just the place where people cook, where they store crockery and pans and their provisions. It is often also where people eat, and where the family gathers for meals. And when friends come to visit, you sit around the kitchen table with them. But the kitchen is also the room where the rubbish bin is, and the recyling bucket is under the sink until someone carries it out. It is also the room where any dirt shows up clearly on the tiled floor. No wonder, then, that we use at least one third of all our household cleaners in the kitchen.

Most people assume that a clean and germ-free kitchen must smell of cleaning agents. Not true! That 'clean' smell only signals that the kitchen is chemically contaminated. And not just the kitchen itself. There are often traces of detergent or rinse aid left on the dishes, residues of scouring powder or disinfectants on work surfaces, and a touch of aggressive fat solvents in the saucepans. If you read the list of ingredients in the detergents found in an average kitchen, you probably won't even know what most of them are. And you probably wouldn't be pleased if you

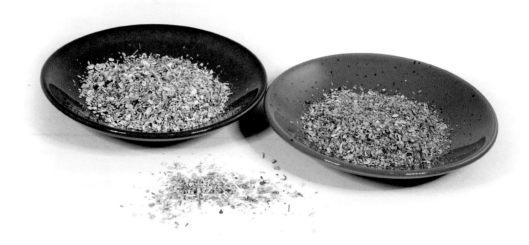

knew. In order to keep a kitchen clean, it is not necessary to compromise your health and spend a lot of household money on a huge amount of industrial cleaning chemicals.

We can produce all the cleaning products we need for the kitchen ourselves. It is simple, cheap and safe for our health. And we aren't just talking about our grandmothers' detergent recipes. Everything that a modern, high-tech kitchen needs in terms of cleaning products, whether for cleaning the microwave, fridge or the oven, to making powder for the dishwasher and descaler for the coffee machine – it can all be made by you.

SOME GENERAL TIPS

While they are still fresh, grease splashes in the oven should be sprinkled with salt. Then as soon as the oven has cooled down, you can simply wipe it all away without leaving any residue.

WOODEN CHOPPING BOARDS look good, but are difficult to clean. It is easier if you rub the dry boards with the cut surface of half a lemon. The oil in the lemon skin will help counteract any grease. You can also use the antibacterial effect of lemon with the fat-dissolving power of essential citrus oil: soak the boards in lukewarm water, to which you add 10-15 drops of this fragrant fat solvent and bacteria killer, based on about five litres of water in the sink. After two to three hours, rinse hot, and the chopping boards will look – and smell – like new!

Something boiling over cannot always be avoided. The outline of burnt-on material on **CERAMIC HOBS** is easier to remove if sprinkled with a little salt while still just warm. Then wipe away using a cloth moistened with vinegar.

If you place casserole dishes in the oven on a **BAKING TRAY** rather than on a rack, spillage due to overflowing will be less of a problem. Cleaning a baking tray is much easier than cleaning the bottom of the oven.

Baked or even **BURNT-ON LEFTOVERS** on saucepans and casserole dishes can be loosened more easily if you sprinkle some washing soda over the leftovers and leave the pot or pan to stand for quarter of an hour. Then mix three tablespoons washing soda in a cup of water, pour into the casserole dish or pan and bring to the boil briefly. After the soda solution has cooled down, the residues can usually simply be rinsed off.

The **DRAIN OF THE KITCHEN SINK** has a lot to cope with, from greasy washing up water to bits of leftover food. No wonder it's prone to constipation! You can counteract this tendency by pouring coffee grounds down the plug into the drain from time to time and rinsing them away with plenty of hot water. This removes greasy residues from the u-bend and drain of the sink.

UNPLEASANT ODOURS IN THE FRIDGE, freezer compartment and deep freeze often arise, sometimes for no apparent reason. However, it is usually because some foods give off odours which are absorbed by other food, making the matter worse. A forgotten yoghurt, different types of cheese and even vegetables can be responsible for this smell. To remove it, empty the fridge, turn the temperature control to zero and wipe it out with a soft cloth and a solution of 100ml water, 20g bicarbonate of soda and five drops of essential peppermint oil. Then wipe again with plain water to remove any bicarbonate of soda residues. Before you turn the fridge back on, everything should be wiped dry. The same procedure can also be applied to freezers.

You can also choose how you want your fridge to smell. Simply place a small bowl with your favourite fragrance on the bottom shelf, so it always smells fresh. For example, if you like vanilla fragrance, pour about 50ml of vanilla extract into the bowl. Vanillin – a synthetic vanilla aroma – serves the same purpose. If you like the smell of coffee, you can put ground coffee in the bowl. The fridge then smells discreetly of coffee for several weeks. You can further refine the fragrance by mixing ground spices, such as ginger, with the coffee.

If instead you want a completely odourless fridge, there's a simple way: just put a slice of bread in the bottom compartment! But change this slice of bread every two days, otherwise it will become mouldy and defeat the purpose.

COCKROACHES, ANTS AND OTHER INSECTS find their way into the cleanest kitchen. But there are a number of tried and tested household remedies to spoil their stay. Bicarbonate of soda helps against ants, because strong odours repel them. If ants are running around in the kitchen cupboards, it is best to wipe them out with a solution of 30g bicarbonate of soda in 200ml water. Then wipe with clear water and then again with a solution of ten drops of essential citrus oil per 100ml of water. The kitchen cupboards then smell pleasantly fresh for human noses, but not for ants.

Cockroaches can be dealt with in similar manner. You can also sprinkle washing soda into the cracks and corners where the unwanted guests like to hide.

Silverfish can easily be lured into a trap, because they like sugar. So hollow out a potato, sprinkle sugar in it, cover this 'trap' with a cloth and place it where you last saw silverfish. The next day you will find them trapped and the potato and the silverfish can be removed/disposed of. Their recurrence can largely be prevented by mixing 15 drops of essential lavender oil in 200ml of water, filling this solution into a spray bottle and spraying the marching routes of the silverfish with it. They'll hate it!

WASHING-UP LIQUID

Dishwashing liquids traditionally smell of lemon, lime or orange. This is no coincidence, because essential citrus oil is a powerful fat solvent. And if we hand-make dishwashing liquids ourselves, we have a huge advantage over industrial detergent manufacturers: we can actually use genuine, pure essential citrus oil! And not only that – many herbs have a considerable cleaning power in themselves.

WASHING-UP LIQUID CONCENTRATE WITH LEMON

50g grated curd soap or soap flakes
1 litre water
15 drops essential citrus oil

Put the grated curd soap or the soap flakes into a pan, pour in a litre of water and bring to the boil, stirring continuously. Then remove the pan from the heat and stir until the soap flakes are completely dissolved. Allow to cool, stir in the essential citrus oil and pour into a suitable storage bottle.

This detergent is a concentrate, of which a little is added to the washing-up water.

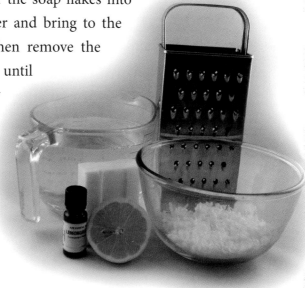

WASHING-UP LIQUID WITH ROSEMARY

100ml pure liquid soap
500ml rosemary decoction
15 drops essential rosemary oil

Pour half a litre of boiling water over two tablespoons of dried rosemary. Allow to steep for about ten minutes, then strain. While still hot, stir in the liquid soap. After cooling, stir in the essential rosemary oil and pour the concentrate into a storage bottle. This washing-up liquid not only smells fresh and vibrant like rosemary, it also has immense fat-dissolving power!

By the way: instead of liquid soap you can of course also boil soap flakes or grated curd soap with water and stir to make your own liquid soap!

WASHING-UP LIQUID WITH FRUIT FRAGRANCE

100ml pure liquid soap
500ml mint extract
20g citric acid
15 drops essential lime oil

Pour a little more than half a litre of boiling water over two tablespoons of dried mint. Allow to steep for about ten minutes, then strain, cool slightly and dissolve the citric acid completely in it by stirring. Then mix with the liquid soap. Finally stir in the essential lime oil (alternatively also citrus oil or lemongrass oil) and pour the fruity fragrant liquid concentrate into a storage bottle. This detergent also has no problem with burnt-on crust!

WASHING-UP LIQUID FOR EXTRA-GREASY DISHES

70g curd soap flakes
1 litre boiling water
30g washing soda
15 drops essential citrus oil

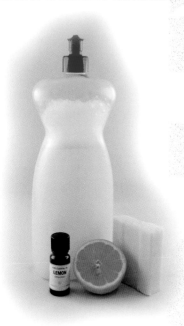

Pour the boiling water over the soap flakes and stir until the soap is completely dissolved. Then add the washing soda and continue stirring until completely dissolved. After cooling, stir in the essential citrus oil and pour the concentrate into a storage bottle. Use as any washing-up liquid. It makes even the greasiest dishes sparkling clean!

SCOURER FOR BURNED-ON FOOD

A powder that can be mixed in advance and stored in a sprinkling container. This simple product significantly reduces the effort of scrubbing the remains of burnt-on food from a pan.

50g washing soda
50g citric acid powder

Mix both ingredients. Sprinkle thoroughly onto burnt-on food in pans and casserole dishes. Then add some warm water and let the pan stand for quarter of an hour. It foams a lot at first, but that shows it's working. The burnt-on material should then be easily removed with a scouring cloth.

GRANDMA'S DETERGENT WITH LEMON SCENT

30g grated curd soap (or soap flakes)
10 drops essential citrus oil
1 litre boiling water
1 teaspoon bicarbonate of soda

This is a detergent recipe that can be found in many post-war household books. The essential lemon oil, however, is a modern addition – Grandma would have managed without.

The soap flakes are covered with boiling water in a sufficiently large jar with a screw cap and completely dissolved by stirring. Allow to cool a little, then stir in the washing soda and finally the essential citrus oil. Leave the jar open until it has cooled to room temperature, then close the lid. After a few hours the soap thickens to a gel. From this concentrate you use about two tablespoons for a sink of dirty dishes.

WASHING-UP LIQUID WITH VINEGAR AND LEMON

You can quickly wash dishes with vinegar in the water. The action of the vinegar dissolves mineral deposits and kills bacteria and germs. But the fat-dissolving power of pure vinegar is limited. This shortcoming can be overcome by using hot water and combining the vinegar with the fat-dissolving power of lemon – either as lemon juice or essential lemon oil.

500ml white vinegar
20 drops essential lemon oil

... are well shaken in a storage bottle. Simply pour the required amount into the hot washing-up water.

GRANDMA'S DETERGENT WITH LEMON SCENT ////////////

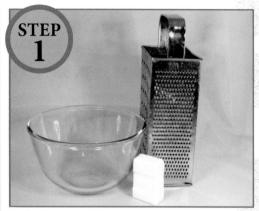

STEP 1

Curd soap, grated. Alternatively you can use soap flakes.

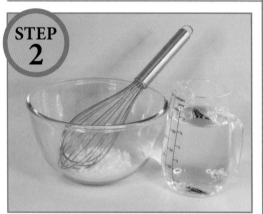

STEP 2

Pour boiling water over it.

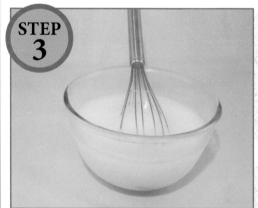

STEP 3

Stir well until the soap is completely dissolved.

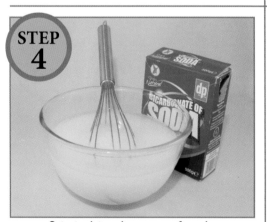

STEP 4

Stir in bicarbonate of soda.

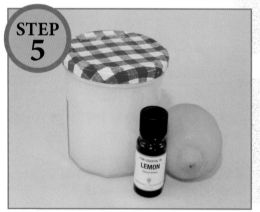

STEP 5

Add essential oil, stir well and leave until cool. Then fill into a screw cap jar.

DISHWASHER POWDER AND RINSE AID

LAVENDER POWDER FOR THE DISHWASHER

When a dishwasher is in use, the kitchen smells of it. And often not particularly pleasant. This dishwasher powder is completely different, allowing a delicate, unobtrusive lavender scent to escape from the dishwasher.

150g bicarbonate of soda
50g salt
50g citric acid powder
15 drops essential lavender oil

Thoroughly mix the sodium bicarbonate, salt (preferably coarse sea salt) and citric acid and put into a sealable plastic container. Sprinkle with the essential lavender oil and mix well. Use two heaped tablespoons of this powder for one cycle.

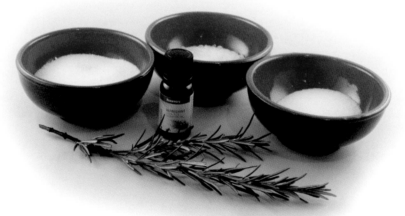

ROSEMARY POWDER FOR THE DISHWASHER

100g washing soda
100g salt
50g citric acid powder
15 drops essential rosemary oil

Washing soda, salt crystals and citric acid powder are mixed thoroughly together and filled into a suitable storage container. Sprinkle the dry mixture with the essential rosemary oil and mix well. Two tablespoons of this powder are enough for a wash, which also cleans heavily soiled dishes and fills the kitchen with a delicate rosemary fragrance.

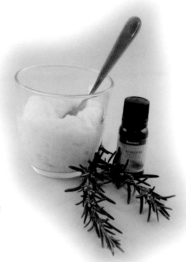

QUICK DISHWASHER POWDER

4 tablespoons bicarbonate of soda
1 tablespoon salt
1 tablespoon citric acid powder

Can be produced quickly when needed: the three powdered ingredients are mixed well together. For one wash cycle, two tablespoons are put into the detergent compartment of the dishwasher. The above quantity is therefore sufficient for three wash cycles.

DISHWASHER POWDER FOR GLASSWARE

100g washing soda
100g bicarbonate of soda
50g citric acid powder
20 drops essential citrus oil

Put all the ingredients in a plastic container and mix well. Add the powder generously to the dishwasher's detergent compartment.

This shiny rinsing powder is particularly suitable for glasses and glass dishes. It ensures shiny cleanliness without leaving water stains on the glass.

CLOVE DISHWASHER POWDER

100g citric acid powder
100g bicarbonate of soda
100g washing soda
50g coarse salt
10 drops essential clove oil

Mix the dry ingredients together well, sprinkle with the essential clove oil, mix thoroughly and store in an airtight container.

RINSE AID WITH ALCOHOL

300ml white vinegar
100ml surgical spirit (70%)

Pour vinegar and alcohol into a bottle, shake well and, when glasses are washed, pour into the rinse-aid compartment of the dishwasher. About two teaspoons 100ml should be sufficient for one cycle. This rinse aid prevents unattractive water stains on the glasses.

You can buy this alcohol in pharmacies and hardware shops. Instead of the one with 70 per cent alcohol content you can also use the one with 96 per cent.

RINSE AID FOR HARD WATER

200ml vinegar essence (20-25%)
300ml distilled water

If unattractive calcium stains are found on cutlery, glasses and glass dishes after rinsing, this is a sign of very hard water. However, you can easily avoid the limescale residues by mixing vinegar essence with distilled water and pouring about 100ml of this mixture into the rinse aid compartment of the dishwasher.

This homemade rinse aid provides a spotless shine!

SCOURING POWDER AND SCOURING CREAM

These scouring agents can be used for sinks and dishes, as well as for worktops and hotplates. Whether as powder or as scouring cream, you can simply make them yourself. And you can use the cleansing power of different herbs. Not only do they smell good, they also act as an abrasive with their hard leaves and the fat dissolving power of their essential oils. Only dried herbs are suitable for use in cleaning agents. These are crushed to a coarse powder in a mortar before use.

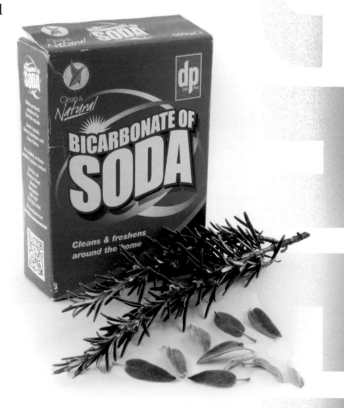

SCOURING POWDER FOR STUBBORN STAINS ///////////////////////////////

100g bicarbonate of soda
20g salt
10 drops essential rosemary or eucalyptus oil
White vinegar for wiping off

Bicarbonate of soda and salt are mixed thoroughly, then sprinkled with the essential rosemary or eucalyptus oil, mixed again and put into an airtight tin. If you have stubborn stains in your stainless steel sink or your stainless steel draining board, sprinkle this powder on top and leave it to work for about quarter of an hour. Then you scrub the surface with a wet sponge, wipe away the residue and then wipe the surface with enough vinegar.

INSTANT SCOURING LIQUID WITH VINEGAR ////////////////////////////

50g bicarbonate of soda
100ml white vinegar
5 drops of essential lavender or citrus oil

Add the soda into the vinegar and completely dissolve by stirring. Then add the essential lavender or citrus oil, stir again and you have an instant scouring agent.

MARIGOLD SCOURING POWDER ///

50g bicarbonate of soda
50g washing soda
30g dried calendula (marigold flowers, coarsely ground)

Bicarbonate of soda, washing soda and dried calendula are mixed thoroughly and placed in a sealable container. This scouring powder is just as suitable for sinks as for worktops and moderately soiled hotplates. Sprinkle it on the surface to be cleaned and scrub it with a damp sponge. Then wipe with pure water to remove any remaining traces.

CINNAMON SCOURING POWDER

100g bicarbonate of soda
20g ground cinnamon
10 drops essential cedar oil

Bicarbonate of soda and cinnamon are mixed, then sprinkled with the essential cedar oil and mixed again thoroughly. The powder is then placed in an airtight container. This scouring powder is particularly suitable for greasy dirt. Sprinkle the powder on the dirty surface, scrub with a wet sponge, wipe with water and then dry, so that there are no residues of the soda left on the surface.

SCOURING POWDER WITH SAGE AND ROSEMARY

100g bicarbonate of soda
20g dried sage leaves, coarsely ground
20g dried rosemary leaves, coarsely
    ground

Bicarbonate of soda and the ground herbs are placed in an airtight container and shaken well so that all the ingredients mix thoroughly. This scouring powder is particularly suitable for sinks. Pour a small amount of it into the basin and scrub it clean with a wet sponge. The residue is washed away with hot water.

SCOURING POWDER WITH MINT AND LEMON BALM

100g bicarbonate of soda
10g coarse salt
20g dried, coarsely ground peppermint
20g dried, coarsely ground lemon balm

Put all ingredients in a sealable box and shake vigorously so that they blend fully. This scouring powder is a universal agent, which can be used for either greasy sinks, hobs or the kitchen floor.

SCOURING POWDER WITH THYME

50g bicarbonate of soda
50g washing soda
30g dried, coarsely ground thyme

Bicarbonate of soda, washing soda and ground thyme are thoroughly mixed and filled into a sealable container. This scouring powder is suitable for sinks, worktops and moderately soiled hotplates. Spread it on the surface to be cleaned and scrub it with a damp sponge. Then rinse with water to remove any remaining traces.

SCOURING CREAM WITH ROSEMARY

30g dried rosemary
100ml boiling water
100g salt
100g washing soda

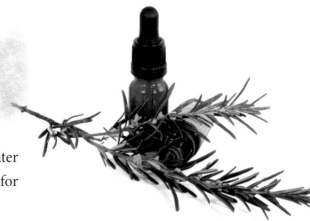

Pour a little more than 100ml boiling water over the dried rosemary, leave to stand for about 15 minutes, then strain to remove the rosemary. Mix washing soda and salt and add spoonfuls to the rosemary liquid and stir in until a paste with a gel-like consistency is obtained.

This scouring paste can also be produced in larger quantities for stock and stored in suitable, well-sealed containers. It is suitable for worktops, hotplates and sinks. After scrubbing with a wet sponge, wipe thoroughly with water to remove the last traces of salt and soda.

SCRUBBING CREAM WITH SALT AND SAGE

100g salt
20g dried, finely ground sage
100ml boiling water
50g bicarbonate of soda
10 drops essential sage oil

Pour the boiling water over the dried, finely ground sage and let it steep for about ten minutes. Do not strain! Allow to cool a little, then stir in salt and bicarbonate of soda and continue stirring until both have dissolved completely. After cooling to room temperature, stir in the essential sage oil and pour into a bottle.

Small amounts of this powerful scouring cream are sufficient to clean even heavily soiled and greasy surfaces. After scrubbing with a wet sponge, wipe with water to remove any traces.

SCRUBBING CREAM WITH THYME

30g dried, finely ground thyme
150ml boiling water
150ml liquid soap
30g washing soda
10 drops essential thyme oil

The dried and finely ground thyme is tipped into a suitable bowl containing the boiling water. Allow to infuse for ten minutes, do not strain, but stir in the liquid soap. As soon as this forms an even solution with the thyme extract, stir in the soda and continue stirring until it has completely dissolved. After cooling, stir in the essential thyme oil and pour the scouring cream into a storage bottle.

With a little scrubbing, this scouring cream also dissolves stubborn and greasy stains. After wiping away with water, a delicate thyme scent remains on the shining surface.

SCOURING CREAM WITH HERBS ///////////////////////////////

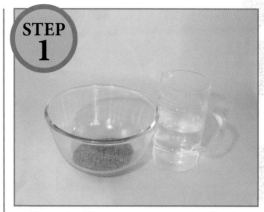

STEP 1

Pour boiling water over the finely chopped herbs and leave to stand.

STEP 2

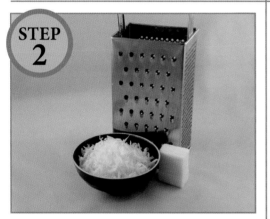

Grate the curd soap to flakes...

STEP 3

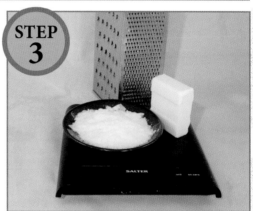

Weigh 40g of curd flakes.

STEP 4

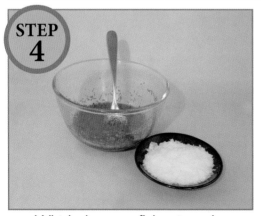

Whisk the soap flakes into the herbal decoction.

STEP 5

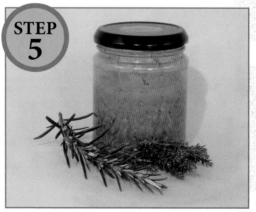

Decant into a bottle.

SCOURING CREAM WITH HERBS

40g grated curd soap or soap flakes
20g dried, finely ground rosemary
20g dried, finely ground thyme
300ml boiling water

Pour boiling water over the finely ground herbs. Allow to steep for about ten minutes. Either grate the curd soap into flakes or weigh out ready-made soap flakes. Then boil the herbal decoction again briefly and stir in the soap flakes. Remove from the heat and stir until the soap has completely dissolved. The fine herb particles are left in the scouring cream. They increase the friction during scrubbing and therefore the effectiveness of the scouring cream.

After cooling to room temperature, the scouring cream is poured into a suitable bottle. It leaves a delicate herbal scent.

YOGHURT SCOURING MILK

100g ground almonds
50ml plain yoghurt
30g washing soda

Sounds like a delicious recipe, but it is intended for scrubbing after cooking! Mix ground almonds and washing soda in yoghurt to a paste. This is rubbed with a damp sponge on the surface to be cleaned until the last trace of dirt has disappeared. Then wipe thoroughly with water.

OVEN CLEANER

In every supermarket you will find a whole shelf of oven cleaners that try to outdo each other in terms of cleaning power. The same applies to the unpleasant and harmful chemicals they contain, because oven cleaners are among the chemical front-runners. Because their traces can never be completely removed from the oven, they continue to burn there as you bake your next cake. This not only smells awful, but the pollutants contained in the smoke of the burnt chemicals can also accumulate in your cake. Reason enough, therefore, to make your own cleaning agents for the oven.

But you'll still have to scrub. The oven is not as easy to clean as a flat work surface. If burnt and encrusted food gathers on the side walls and the bottom of the oven, then only scrubbing will remove it. Even our homemade oven cleaners are not miracle cures that can remove encrusted food without at least *some* scrubbing.

A heavily soiled oven is easier to clean if it is heated to 50°C before cleaning. The heat is then switched off, racks and baking trays are removed and the cleaning paste is spread evenly over the side walls, floor and any dirty areas on the rear wall using a sponge. Because there are fans, lighting and heating elements on the rear wall, appropriate care must be taken there. There may also be ventilation slots on the floor. These should be covered with aluminium foil. Let the paste work for about half an hour and then wipe it off with a scouring cloth. If the encrustations are very stubborn, you may have to scrub a little. Extensive wiping with a sponge and water is necessary to remove all traces of the cleaning paste.

CLEANING PASTE FOR A HEAVILY SOILED OVEN

100g salt
50g washing soda
300g bicarbonate of soda
100ml water
100ml white vinegar
10 drops essential citrus oil

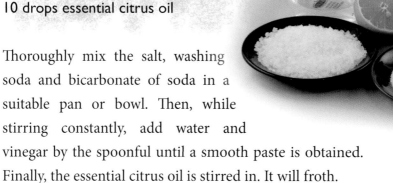

Thoroughly mix the salt, washing soda and bicarbonate of soda in a suitable pan or bowl. Then, while stirring constantly, add water and vinegar by the spoonful until a smooth paste is obtained. Finally, the essential citrus oil is stirred in. It will froth.

SIMPLE SPRAY CLEANER FOR THE OVEN

100g washing soda
100ml liquid soap
100ml water

Mix the liquid soap and water, stir in washing soda and continue stirring until completely dissolved. This liquid cleaner is filled into a spray bottle and sprayed onto the walls and bottom of the oven. After a contact time of about a quarter of an hour, the dirt can be wiped off. Then wipe with water to remove any soap and soda residue.

This simple cleaner works particularly well if the oven is heated to a temperature of about 50°C before cleaning, and then switched off.

TWO-PHASE OVEN CLEANER

100ml vinegar essence
200ml water
10 drops essential citrus oil
30g salt
100g bicarbonate of soda
30ml liquid soap

For the first phase of this cleaner for a heavily soiled oven, mix the vinegar essence with the water and essential citrus oil. This liquid goes into a spray bottle. Spray it on the walls and the bottom of the oven, then repeat the spraying 15 minutes later.

For the second phase, salt, bicarbonate of soda and liquid soap are mixed with a few spoonfuls of water to form a paste. As soon as the spray from phase one has dried a little, spread this paste on the walls and the bottom of the oven and let it work for a few hours. Then wipe it clean with a wet cloth. Thorough wiping with water is necessary to remove all traces of soap and soda.

OVEN CLEANER CONCENTRATE

100g bicarbonate of soda
50g grated curd soap or soap flakes
250ml boiling water
15 drops essential citrus oil

Put grated curd soap or soap flakes in a bowl or pan then pour over with boiling water and stir until the soap has completely dissolved. Then stir in the bicarbonate of soda.

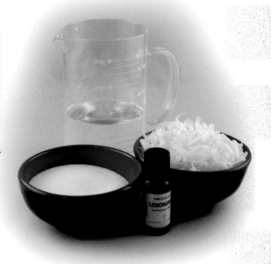

When dissolved and after cooling, add the essential citrus oil. This concentrate is filled into a storage bottle. For use, dilute one part mixture with two parts water, pour into a spray bottle and spray onto the walls and bottom of the warm (about 50 °C) oven. After about a quarter of an hour, wipe it – and the dirt – off with a damp cloth. Then wipe clean with water.

This oven cleaner can also be produced in larger quantities. It is useful for moderate soiling of the oven and general oven cleaning after use.

HOTPLATE CLEANER

Those who have an oven with round, black hotplates know how gruelling cleaning them can be. Here is a cleaner you can use on the warm – but not hot! – cooking plates, and it's a lot easier.

100ml liquid soap
50ml hot water
20g bicarbonate of soda
20g salt
10 drops essential citrus oil

Mix liquid soap, bicarbonate of soda and salt with the hot water to a smooth paste and then stir in the essential citrus oil. This cleaning paste can be stored in an airtight plastic container. When required, brush it onto the soiled and just warm hotplate, leave it to work for a while and then wipe it off with a wet sponge. Only if encrustations are heavily burnt on will scouring powder be needed afterwards.

FRIDGE AND MICROWAVE CLEANERS

Fridges and microwave ovens are particularly susceptible to grease and dirt, even in the form of greasy fingerprints on their outer surfaces. Especially in the fridge, unpleasant odours are often found. You should therefore defrost the fridge regularly and wipe it thoroughly with a cleaner. The recipes for the following detergents usually contain essential oils which, in addition to cleanliness, also ensure the greatest possible sterility and a fresh fragrance.

GREASE-DISSOLVING FRIDGE CLEANER

30g grated curd soap or soap flakes
250ml boiling water
20g bicarbonate of soda
10 drops essential rosemary, lavender or citrus oil

Pour boiling water over the soap flakes in a suitable bowl or pan and stir until completely dissolved. Then stir in the soda powder, also until completely dissolved, and finally the essential oil. This cleaner can be filled into a storage or a spray bottle. However, you must shake it well before each use because the soap tends to settle on the bottom. The cleaner is sprayed generously onto the surface to be cleaned or applied with a sponge and left to act for a short time. Then wipe the surfaces with a wet sponge and dry with a cloth. This cleaner is not only suitable for the fridge, but also for all greasy kitchen appliances.

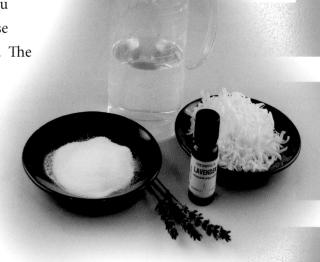

FRIDGE CLEANER WITH ALCOHOL

100ml water
100ml white vinegar
100ml surgical spiritl (70%)
15 drops essential citrus oil

All ingredients are mixed together and filled into a spray bottle. Spray the cleaner on the inside walls, inside the door and on the bottom of the fridge, let it work for a short time and then wipe the surfaces with a wet cloth. This cleaner can also be used to remove dirt from the outside of the fridge door.

FRIDGE CLEANER WITH CITRUS POWER

100ml vinegar essence
approx. 50ml lemon juice
200ml water
20g bicarbonate of soda
10 drops essential citrus oil

Squeeze one or two lemons – you should get about 50ml of liquid – and strain the juice through a coffee filter to remove even the finest fruit flesh residues. Then pour it into a sufficiently large bowl or pan, add the water and stir in the soda powder. When the bicarbonate of soda is completely dissolved, pour the vinegar essence into the solution and stir well again. Finally, stir the essential citrus oil into the solution and pour the cleaner into a spray bottle.

FRIDGE CLEANER WITH SALT

20g salt
300ml boiling water
100ml white vinegar
10 drops of essential peppermint or lemon balm
(melissa) oil

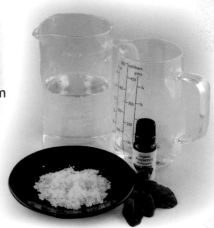

Sprinkle the salt in a suitable container, pour
over the boiling water and dissolve completely
by stirring. Allow to cool a little, then stir in
the vinegar and finally the essential oil. After
cooling, the cleaner is poured into a spray bottle.   It can be sprayed on all internal
and, if necessary, external surfaces of the fridge and wiped with a wet sponge after
a short contact time.

This cleaner can also be used to defrost the freezer compartment. In this case the
essential oil is omitted. Bring the rest to the boil, pour the solution into a wide bowl
and place it in the switched-off freezer compartment. The rising vapours quickly
dissolve the ice and traces of dirt. Check first that you can put hot water in the freezer.

MICROWAVE CLEANER WITH VINEGAR

50g bicarbonate of soda
50ml vinegar essence
100ml water
10 drops essential thyme or citrus oil

Mix water and vinegar essence together, then stir in the soda powder until
completely dissolved. Then the essential thyme or citrus oil is stirred in. Pour into
a spray bottle and spray on the inside of the microwave, avoiding the mechanical

parts – fan, coupling for turntable, ventilation slot. Leave briefly, then wipe the interior with a damp sponge and dry with a cloth. The turntable should be removed before all this and cleaned separately. And always make sure that the mains plug of the appliance is disconnected from the socket during cleaning.

MICROWAVE CLEANING PASTE

100g bicarbonate of soda
1-2 tablespoons vinegar
10 drops essential citrus oil

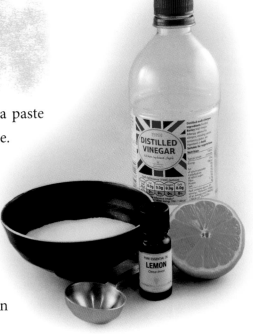

The bicarbonate of soda is stirred into a paste by adding the vinegar one spoon at a time. Then stir in the essential citrus oil. After removing the power plug and the turntable, this paste is applied to the inner surfaces of the microwave. Let them dry a little and then wipe them off with a damp sponge. Wipe dry with a cloth so that no bicarbonate of soda remains in the microwave.

This cleaning paste is particularly suitable for removing unpleasant odours from the microwave or for generally refreshing it.

SALT PASTE FOR THE MICROWAVE

100g bicarbonate of soda
50g salt
100ml hot water
10 drops essential citrus oil

Bicarbonate of soda and salt are mixed and stirred into a thick paste by adding hot water spoon by spoon. Lastly, the essential citrus oil is stirred in. Disconnect the power and remove the turntable, then apply the paste to the inner surfaces of the microwave, avoiding all mechanical parts. Allow the paste to work briefly and then wipe it off with a damp cloth. Wipe with a wet sponge and then dry.

This cleaning paste is particularly effective against burnt-on residues, often found on the side walls and bottom of the microwave.

SPRAY CLEANER WITH SPECIAL GREASE DISSOLVING POWER

40g soap flakes
250ml boiling water
20g bicarbonate of soda
20g salt
10 drops essential citrus oil

Pour the boiling water over the soap flakes in a suitable bowl and stir until completely dissolved. Mix the bicarbonate of soda and salt together and stir into the soap solution. When completely dissolved, stir in the essential citrus oil and pour the cleaner into a spray bottle. It is particularly important to shake thoroughly before use with this cleaner, because the dissolved substances can settle on the bottom of the bottle.

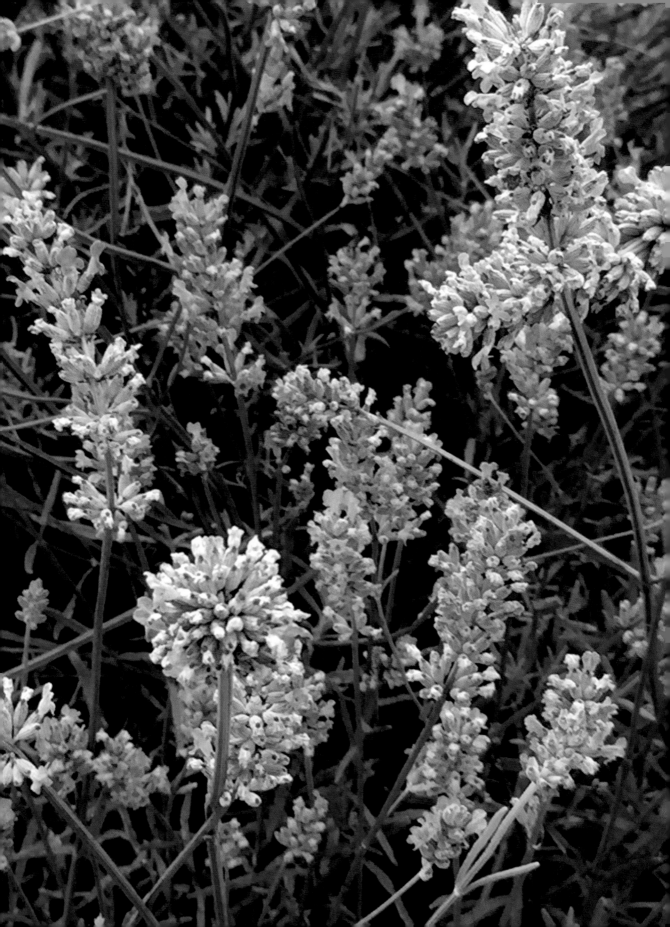

CHAPTER FOUR

THE BATHROOM

PARTICULARLY HIGH STANDARDS OF CLEANLINESS AND HYGIENE ARE NEEDED IN THE BATHROOM. THESE REQUIREMENTS CAN BE MET WITH HOMEMADE CLEANING AND DISINFECTING AGENTS

HYGIENE WITH A FRESH FRAGRANCE

After the kitchen, bathrooms and toilets are the rooms on which we place the highest demands in terms of cleanliness and hygiene. It's where we use most cleaning agents. The bathroom is given this special attention for good reason. Its very purpose makes it a breeding ground for bacteria and mould. You wash there, brush your teeth, comb your hair, rub away dead skin cells. The air humidity of the bathroom is high. And sometimes the bathroom also houses the washing machine and perhaps a tumble dryer, both of which increase humidity.

The most important measure is to ventilate the bathroom thoroughly. But mould and mildew can still find a way to settle there, so appropriate cleaning and disinfection is necessary. The good news is that you don't need to do a massive supermarket chemical blitz. There are a number of cleaning and disinfecting agents that can be produced easily, inexpensively and in a health-friendly way. Optimum cleanliness and hygiene in bathrooms and toilets do *not* depend on industrially-manufactured products – it's just a matter of knowing what to use!

Some well-tried methods help to keep the cleaning effort to a minimum and you'll still have a clean and fresh-smelling bathroom without much effort.

You can get a **FRESH SCENT** in the bathroom by dripping a few drops of an essential oil onto the cardboard tube inside the toilet roll. Choose your favourite essential oil and every time you use toilet paper, the roll moves and the scent spreads throughout the room.

COMBS AND BRUSHES are used every day, so the hair and dead skin cells that accumulate between bristles and teeth should be removed regularly. If necessary, you can put the combs and brushes in a container of 50 per cent vinegar and 50 per cent water, plus a few drops of essential tea tree or eucalyptus oil – this ensures both sterility and a fresh fragrance. After about half an hour take combs and brushes out, clean them with an old toothbrush and rinse them with water.

A fresh atmosphere in the bathroom or toilet does not need to come from chemicals. A **POTPOURRI** will do the job naturally. It's just a bowl in which you put aromatic herbs. Fresh herbs only keep their scent briefly, which is why it is better to use dried herbs and 'scent' them with a few drops of their own essential oil. A potpourri releases its scent for one to two weeks. You can add fresh flowers to the herbs, and thus turn the scent bowl into a very decorative item!

BATH MATS AND TOILET MATS need frequent washing, but you can increase the interval between washes if you occasionally give them a quick clean. Add a few drops of any essential oil to a cup of bicarbonate of soda, mix well and sprinkle the mats with this powder. After half an hour the powder is simply vacuumed off with a vacuum cleaner.

BLOCKED DRAINS from washbasins, shower trays and bathtubs can be cleared with washing soda and boiling water. Sprinkle the washing soda into the drain and slowly pour the boiling water over it until the powder has completely dissolved. Let it work for a while, then rinse thoroughly with water – great fun when you hear the bubbling of the now-clear drain!

DISINFECTANTS

Disinfectants should not only kill off bacteria and germs, but also prevent or eliminate fungal spores, mould and mildew. Wooden window frames and shower curtains are particularly susceptible to mould. Sufficient ventilation is therefore important. As far as shower curtains are concerned, they should be made of a material that can withstand machine washing. If they are hung up to dry in the blazing sun after washing, mould and mildew have no chance to settle on them. For all other cases where disinfection is necessary, homemade disinfectants are ideally suited. They eliminate bacteria, germs, fungal spores and, with the addition of the right essential oils, also viruses.

DISINFECTANT SPRAY WITH CEDAR OIL

20g bicarbonate of soda
250ml warm water
15 drops essential cedar oil

The bicarbonate of soda is completely dissolved in warm water by stirring. Then add the essential cedar oil and pour into a spray bottle. This disinfectant spray works just as well as the best from the supermarket shelf, but smells incomparably better. And if you prefer the scent of spruce instead of cedar, then simply use the scent of pine instead of essential cedar oil!

DISINFECTANT SPRAY WITH THYME

250ml boiling water
5 fresh thyme sprigs
30g bicarbonate of soda
10 drops essential thyme oil

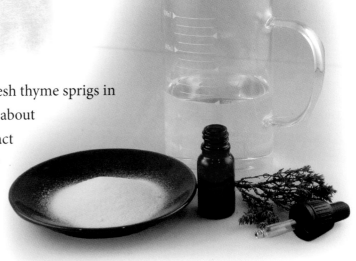

Pour boiling water over the fresh thyme sprigs in
a suitable bowl. Let it steep for about
half an hour, strain the extract
and stir in the soda powder
until completely dissolved.
Then add the essential thyme
oil and transfer the liquid into
a spray bottle. After shaking
the bottle thoroughly, spray this very effective disinfectant onto the surfaces in the
bathroom or toilet and wipe them clean with a damp sponge. You can make a safe
and effective disinfectant spray yourself so simply!

DISINFECTANT SPRAY FOR THE TOILET

100ml white vinegar
150ml surgical spirit
20 drops tea tree oil

All ingredients are mixed together and poured into a spray bottle. This disinfectant
spray can handle bacteria and germs of all kinds and also provides a fresh fragrance.
Because of its intensity, however, it should only be used in small quantities.

MOULD REMOVER

ANTI-MOULD SPRAY

100ml white vinegar essence
100ml water
5 drops essential cinnamon oil
15 drops essential tea tree oil

All ingredients are mixed together and filled into a spray bottle. Spray this effective mould killer on any mould stains on the wall or other areas affected by mould. You don't wipe it off, you let it dry on. Only after a few hours do you wipe with a soft cloth and repeat the process, but without wiping after drying.

MOULD KILLER WITH ALCOHOL

100ml surgical spirit (70%)
100ml water
5 drops essential thyme oil
10 drops essential tea tree oil

Mix all ingredients together and fill into a spray bottle. Spray on areas affected by mould, allow to dry and repeat this process several times. You can spray these mould killers in joints and cracks and let them dry there. However, care must be taken to avoid rubber seals and plastic parts because they can deteriorate due to the alcohol.

ANTI-MOULD SPRAY

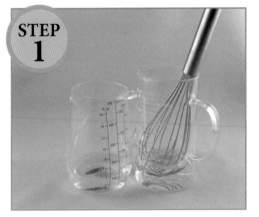

STEP 1

Mix vinegar essence with water.

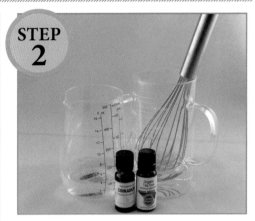

STEP 2

Stir in the essential oil.

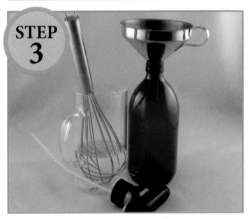

STEP 3

Pour into a spray bottle.

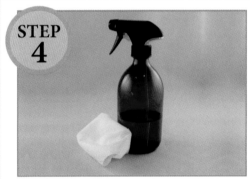

STEP 4

Spray the mould stain with the spray and wipe with a soft cloth. Repeat the procedure several times, do not wipe after the last time, but allow to dry.

SPRAY AGAINST MOULD AND MILDEW

250ml water
10 drops citrus seed extract
10 drops essential tea tree oil

Citrus seed extract and tea tree oil are mixed in the water and filled into a spray bottle. This disinfectant is ideal for the prevention of mould and mildew. It is sprayed onto all areas of the bathroom where condensation forms, from the bathroom cabinet door to the shower curtain and into all joints and cracks. This mixture is sprayed in large quantities onto the appropriate areas and is not wiped off afterwards. Simply leave to dry by good ventilation in the room.

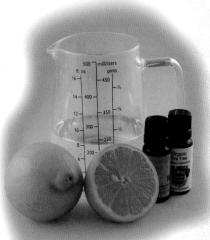

UNIVERSAL BATHROOM CLEANER

To protect particularly sensitive surfaces, such as marble, the normal all-purpose cleaner is not suitable. Here a mild bath cleaner is used which reliably removes dirt and limescale deposits.

MILD UNIVERSAL CLEANER FOR THE BATHROOM

150ml white vinegar
20ml coconut surfactant
100ml water
10 drops essential lavender oil

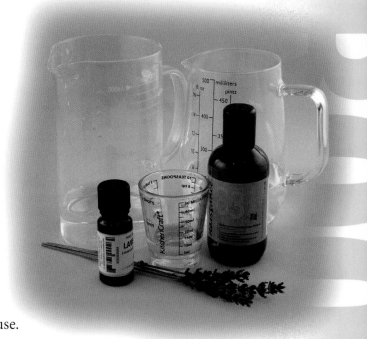

Bring the water to the boil and stir in the coconut surfactant. Allow to cool a little, then stir in the vinegar and finally the essential lavender oil. This cleaner is very thin so it works well in a spray bottle. Because the coconut surfactant tends to settle on the bottom, you should shake the spray bottle well before each use.

Coconut surfactant is a pure natural product, which can be bought cheaply in chemists, health food shops and online.

MIRROR CLEANER

A good mirror cleaner removes dirt without leaving streaks. It also has the bonus that the mirror no longer fogs up; it is a pure miracle weapon.

QUICK MIRROR CLEANER

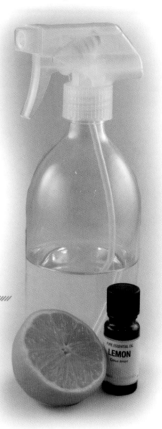

100ml white vinegar
200ml distilled water
50ml surgical spirit
10 drops essential eucalyptus oil

All ingredients are mixed together and filled into a spray bottle. The cleaner is sprayed onto the mirror, wiped off and it shines with streak-free cleanliness.

MIRROR CLEANER WITH ANTI-MIST

100ml vinegar essence
150ml water
10 drops essential citrus oil

All ingredients are mixed together and filled into a spray bottle. Shake well before use, then spray on and wipe with a dry cloth. This cleaner has the side effect that mirrors cleaned with it no longer mist up with steam from the shower cubicle.

SCOURING POWDER AND CREAMS

For everything that needs scrubbing, the scouring agents recommended as kitchen cleaners are suitable to use in the bathroom. However, because there is such emphasis on antibacterial and disinfectant properties in bathrooms and toilets, and because bathrooom scouring agents also need a fresh herbal fragrance, here are a number of scouring agent recipes especially for bathrooms and toilets.

SCRUBBING POWDER WITH HERBS

100g bicarbonate of soda
20g dried sage leaves
20g dried rosemary leaves
1 heaped teaspoon of cream of tartar

The dried sage and rosemary leaves are ground to a coarse powder in a mortar, then mixed with bicarbonate of soda and cream of tartar and placed in a suitable container, preferably one suitable for sprinkling. The scouring powder is sprinkled in washbasins, bathtubs or shower trays. Scrub with a wet cloth or sponge and rinse well with water. The coarse particles of the herbs increase not only the cleaning power of the cleaner, but also the friction between cloth and dirt.

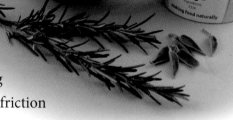

SCOURING POWDER WITH ROSEMARY

100g bicarbonate of soda
100g washing soda
30g dried rosemary leaves
10 drops essential rosemary oil

The dried rosemary leaves are ground to a coarse powder in a pestle and mortar, mixed well with bicarbonate of soda and washing soda and finally sprinkled with the essential rosemary oil. Mix the whole thing again well and pour into a container, preferably one with a sprinkling lid. The scouring powder is spread on the surface to be cleaned, then scrubbed with a wet cloth or sponge and rinsed thoroughly with water.

SCOURING POWDER FOR STAINS

150g bicarbonate of soda
1 heaped teaspoon of wine stone baking powder
zest of two lemons

Grated lemon zest, bicarbonate of soda and the baking powder are mixed well and filled into a suitable container. The scouring powder is scattered on the surface to be cleaned, then scrubbed and finally rinsed with water. This powder is particularly effective against stubborn stains and has a mild bleaching effect.

SCOURING POWDER FOR
GREASE AND SOAP RESIDUE

100g washing soda
100g bicarbonate of soda
50g salt

All ingredients are mixed well together and filled into a suitable container, preferably one with a sprinkler. You put the scouring powder on a wet sponge or cloth and scrub the sink or bathtub with it. This scouring powder dissolves greasy dirt and soap residues particularly well. Thorough rinsing with water will remove all traces of the powder from the drain.

FOAMING SCOURING POWDER

100g bicarbonate of soda
5 drops essential lemon oil
100ml white vinegar

The bicarbonate of soda is well mixed with the essential lemon oil. Sprinkle this scouring powder into the sink and pour the vinegar over it. This should now foam vigorously. As soon as it stops, wipe the sink clean with a wet sponge or cloth and rinse with water.

DISINFECTANT SCOURING POWDER WITH LEMON

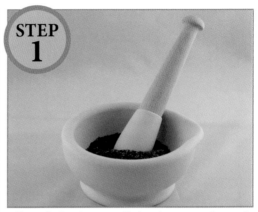

STEP 1

Grind the lemon balm in a pestle and mortar to a coarse powder.

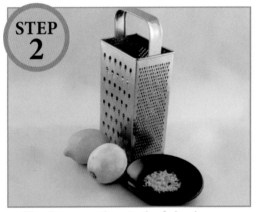

STEP 2

Finely grate the rind of the lemon.

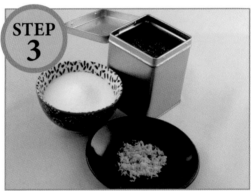

STEP 3

Mix lemon balm, lemon zest and bicarbonate of soda in a biscuit or coffee tin.

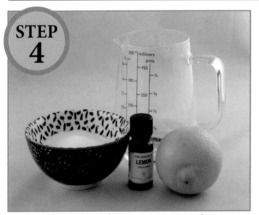

STEP 4

Sprinkle the mixture with essential oil ...

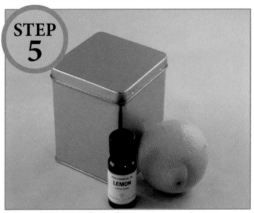

STEP 5

... and shake vigorously.

DISINFECTANT SCOURING POWDER WITH LEMON //////////////

150g bicarbonate of soda
30g dried lemon balm leaves
zest of a lemon
15 drops essential citrus oil

The dried leaves of the lemon balm are ground in a pestle and mortar to a coarse powder, mixed with the bicarbonate of soda and zest of a lemon, then sprinkled with the essential citrus oil. Mix well and store in an airtight container. The scouring powder is spread on the surface to be cleaned, scrubbed with a wet cloth or sponge and then rinsed thoroughly with water. Not only is the sink or bath clean, but bacteria and germs are eliminated and disposed of down the drain. This scouring agent has an immense antibacterial and germicidal effect!

DISINFECTANT SCOURING POWDER WITH ROSEMARY //////////

100g bicarbonate of soda
100g washing soda
30g dried rosemary leaves
15 drops essential rosemary oil

The dried rosemary leaves are ground to a coarse powder in a mortar. Then mix the powder with bicarbonate of soda and washing soda and sprinkle the mixture with the essential rosemary oil. Mix well so that the essential oil comes into contact with all the powder, then pour into an airtight container.

This scouring powder smells like a garden. And the crushed rosemary leaves improve the scrubbing effect enormously!

GENTLE SCOURING PASTE WITH LAVENDER

150g bicarbonate of soda
50g dried milk powder
100ml liquid curd soap
10 drops essential lavender oil
some water

Bicarbonate of soda and dried milk powder are mixed in the liquid curd soap. Then mix in the essential lavender oil and continue stirring with a little water until a smooth paste is obtained. Then pour into a suitable bottle. This gentle scouring agent should be sufficient for all cleaning needs in bathrooms and toilets. And, of course, there is nothing to stop you from making the liquid curd soap yourself from soap flakes or grated solid curd soap.

SCRUBBING PASTE FOR BATHS, SINKS AND TILES

150ml liquid soap
50g bicarbonate of soda
5 drops essential tea tree or eucalyptus oil
some water

Mix the liquid soap and bicarbonate of soda in a suitable bowl, stir in the essential oil and continue stirring, adding spoonfuls of water as required, until a smooth, rather thin paste is obtained. Store in a sealed bottle. The paste is applied to the surfaces of the bathtub or tiles and rubbed with a wet sponge or cloth until the surfaces are clean. Rinse or wipe with water to remove all soap residue.

SCRUB PASTE WITH SALT AND VINEGAR

100g bicarbonate of soda
100g coarse salt
10 drops essential citrus oil
some white vinegar

Bicarbonate of soda, salt and essential citrus oil are well mixed in a suitable bowl. Then add the vinegar by the spoonful and stir until you have a smooth paste. Careful, it foams vigorously when the vinegar meets the natron salt and the soda mixture! It is best to wait until the foam has calmed down a little before stirring.

This scouring paste is particularly suitable for bathtubs and washbasins.

ANTISEPTIC TOILET CLEANER

A thorough clean, which also destroys germs, is particularly important in the toilet. This does not only concern the toilet bowl itself. This is actually a relatively clean place. Most bacteria and germs can be found on the underside of the seat and in the area around the hinges. Since toilet lids and flush-handles or buttons are often touched, this area should not only be cleaned, but also disinfected frequently. The ideal solution, of course, is a cleaning agent that performs these two tasks in one wipe. The adverts for industrially-produced WC cleaners are full of promises in this respect. But we needn't be impressed, because our homemade toilet cleaners can do the job just as well. And that's without leaving behind a chemically-contaminated 'smallest room'.

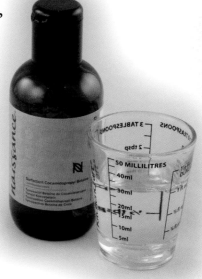

CLEANING SPRAY FOR THE TOILET /////////

100ml water
100ml white vinegar
30ml coconut surfactant
15 drops essential tea tree oil

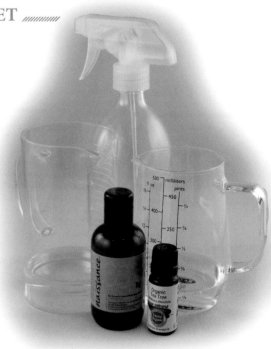

Pour a good 100ml of boiling water over the surfactant in a bowl and dissolve it completely by stirring. Allow to cool a little, then stir in the vinegar and the essential tea tree oil. Decant into a spray bottle.

This practical cleaning spray is ready for regular cleaning of the entire toilet.

ANTIBACTERIAL TOILET SPRAY //

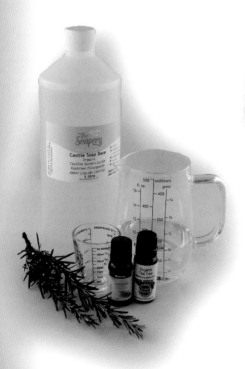

50ml liquid soap (liquid curd
        or Castile liquid soap)
200ml hot water
15 drops essential tea tree oil
10 drops of essential eucalyptus or rosemary oil

In a mixing bowl, add the liquid soap and the hot water in a suitable bowl and stir until completely dissolved. Then add the essential oils and pour into a spray bottle.

Due to its concentrated antibacterial effect, this spray is particularly suitable for cleaning the toilet seat and its underside. In the toilet bowl it eliminates all micro-organisms.

TOILET BOWL CLEANER

100g bicarbonate of soda
100ml white vinegar
10 drops of essential cedar or pine oil
10 drops essential citrus oil

Slowly and carefully pour the vinegar over the soda powder in a suitable glass bowl. It foams violently – as always when vinegar meets bicarbonate of soda. When things have calmed down a little, stir well until the soda powder is completely dissolved in the vinegar. Finally, the essential oils are stirred in and the cleaner is stored in an airtight bottle.

This cleaner removes stubborn rings and discolorations in the toilet bowl. It is poured onto the inside of the toilet bowl and left to work overnight. In the morning it is usually sufficient to flush the toilet and the discolorations or rings are gone.

POWERFUL URINE STAIN REMOVER

100g salt
50g washing soda
50g citric acid powder
50g tartaric acid powder

All dry ingredients are mixed together throughly and stored in a tin. When required, sprinkle this powder into the toilet bowl and scrub away all deposits with the brush. This powder has a gentle bleaching effect so that discolorations can be easily removed.

FRAGRANCE SPRAY
FOR THE TOILET

There are often smells in the toilet, that's the nature of things. Many room sprays from the supermarket only mask the odour with a different, synthetic aroma. The following natural fragrance spray is not only pleasant, it is also able to bind to the unpleasant odours and actually removes them from the room air.

200ml lavender water
10 drops essential lavender oil
10 drops essential rosemary oil

Lavender water is made by placing fresh stems of lavender in a wide bowl and pouring water over them – ideally distilled water, but that's not essential. Cover with a glass lid or a flat glass pane and place it in the blazing sun for a whole sunny day. Whenever you move the bowl to a new, sunny place, check the water level and top it up if necessary. By evening you will have water smelling lightly but beautifully of lavender. It contains not only the essential oils of the plant, but also a whole range of other elements that are useful as odour binders.

To make the fragrance stronger, add essential lavender and rosemary oil to the lavender water, then pour into a spray bottle. When required, spray once or twice into the air, and the toilet will be fragrant – in a good way.

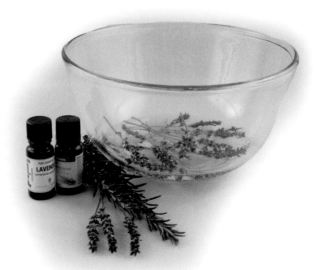

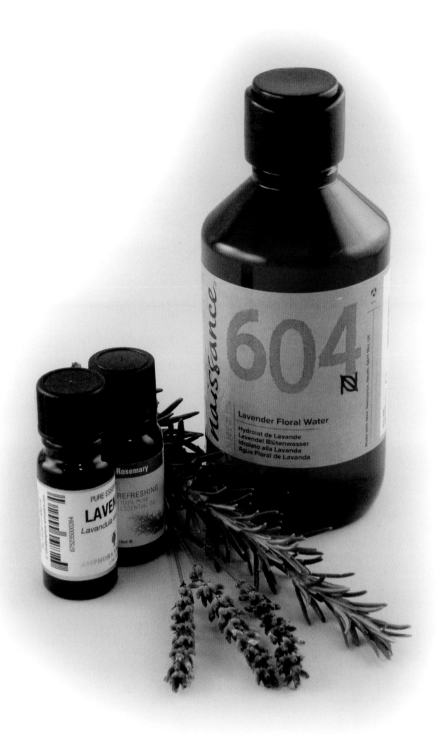

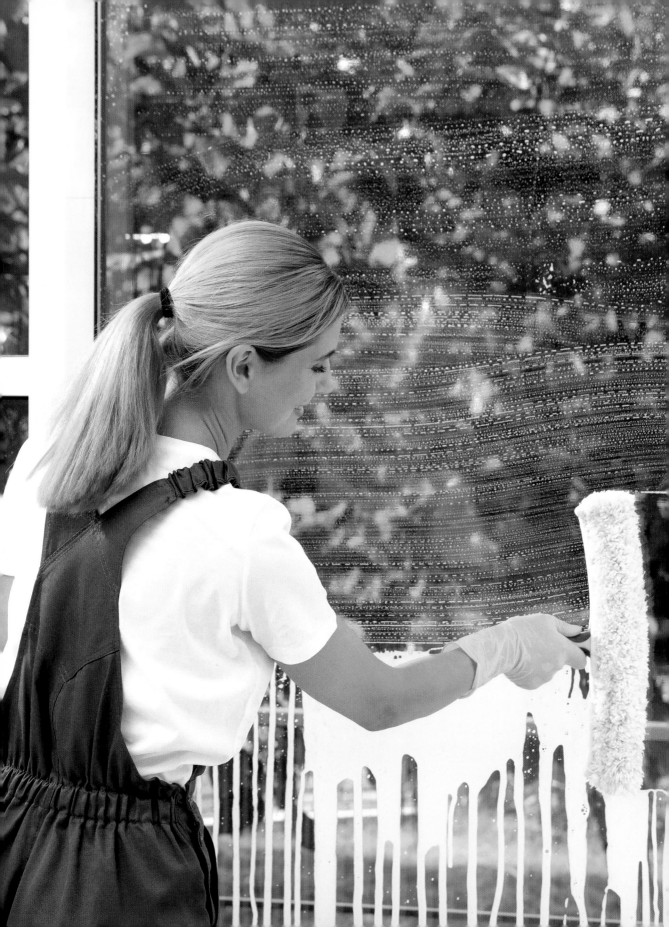

CHAPTER FIVE

WINDOWS

THE WINDOWS CONNECT YOUR LIVING SPACE WITH THE OUTSIDE WORLD

It isn't easy to clean window panes without leaving streaks. And depending on whether you live in the country or the city, or on a busy road, your windows will require cleaning at shorter or longer intervals. And cleaned windows don't stay streak free and shiny for very long. Supermarket window cleaning products often contain substances of concern, including volatile organic compounds such as glycol ethers.

Soft leather cloths are the traditional tools for cleaning window panes. A leather cloth is simply moistened, and the window surface is wiped with it. Always from top to bottom, never across. The leather cloth should always be clean and wrung out during the process. So you have to rinse it out frequently in clear water and wring it out well. A soft cotton window cloth is

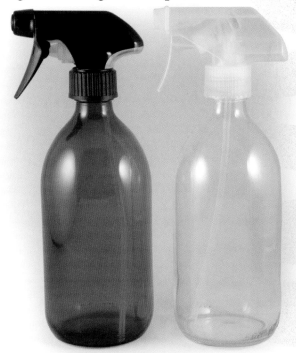

more suitable than a leather cloth for the final removal of individual water droplets.

Very practical and time-saving are window wiper-blades with a narrow rubber lip, which are also used for cleaning the car windscreen. The window pane is sprayed with cleaning agent, or heavily soiled panes can first be wiped off with a sponge moistened with cleaning agent. Then you always remove the water with the wiper from top to bottom, starting in the upper left corner of the window.

As with many household tasks, there are traditional rules for window cleaning. One of them is that you should never clean windows when the sun is shining on them. It's not clear whether this applies to all methods of window cleaning or only to those involving cloths, sponges and newspaper.

WINDOW CLEANING

Window panes are best polished with a cloth dipped in vinegar. With a second cloth you rub the wet panes dry; with a third cloth you polish them.

Methylated spirit in warm water for window cleaning (about two tablespoons full per bucket) causes faster drying with less tendency to streaking. With methylated spirit you can easily wipe off fly stains from the windows.

Newspaper is not only inexpensive, but also very useful for the final dry polishing of window panes. The printing ink makes the glass shiny.

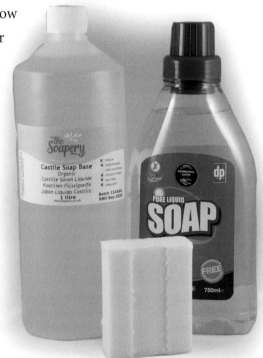

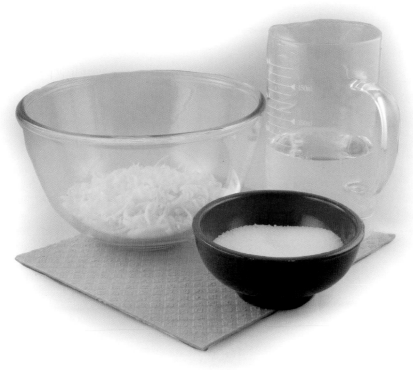

CLEANER FOR HEAVILY SOILED WINDOWS

100g soap flakes or grated curd soap
250ml hot water
50g washing soda

Put the soap flakes in a suitable bowl, add the hot water and stir until completely dissolved. Then stir in washing soda and pour this window cleaning solution into a bottle. Wet a sponge with the cleaner and wipe the window pane. Allow to act briefly, then remove with the wiper-blade.

This cleaner is also suitable for heavily soiled window panes. It easily removes fly droppings and other organic contaminants.

ALL-PURPOSE WINDOW SPRAY

100ml methylated spirit
150ml distilled water
15ml liquid soap
20 drops essential citrus oil

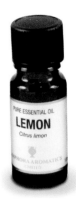

Heat the water a little and fully dissolve the liquid soap by stirring. Then stir in the spirit and finally the essential oil and pour the whole lot into a spray bottle. Then spray on the window panes and clean as usual.

SIMPLE VINEGAR WINDOW SPRAY

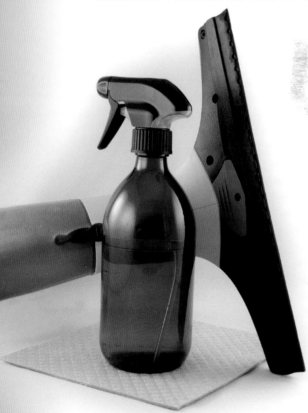

200ml water
100ml white vinegar

This is the classic homemade window cleaner: simply mix vinegar and water thoroughly and pour into a spray bottle. Spray the glass surface with it, remove excess liquid with the wiper-blade, and you're done!

SHINY WINDOWS WITH ANTI-MIST PROTECTION

250ml water
50ml white vinegar essence
20 drops essential citrus oil

The vinegar essence is mixed with the water, then the essential citrus oil is stirred in, and all poured into a spray bottle. This cleaner is particularly suitable for the interior surfaces of bathroom and kitchen windows. The essential oil leaves a wafer-thin film on the glass surface, which prevents misting of the window after showering or steaming in the kitchen.

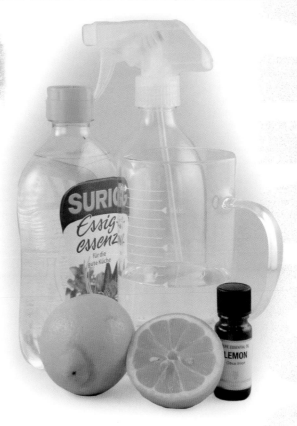

LAUNDRY POWDER

LIQUID DETERGENT
from curd soap
◆ Curd soap ◆ Bicarbonate of soda
◆ Essential oil ◆ Water

ALL-ROUND

MASHING POWDER

CHAPTER SIX

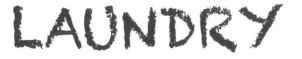

LAUNDRY

THE WASHING MACHINE DOES TODAY WHAT USED TO BE A STRENUOUS JOB. BUT ALL TOO OFTEN A CHEMICAL COCKTAIL IS USED IN THE WASH WHICH DOES OUR SKIN NO GOOD AT ALL. THERE'S ANOTHER WAY.

DO THE LAUNDRY WITHOUT CHLORINE BLEACH, WITHOUT OPTICAL BRIGHTENERS, WITHOUT NANOPARTICLES

We are so dazzled by the advertising of the detergent industry that we can hardly believe it's possible: doing the laundry without industrially-produced washing powder or liquid detergent, without fabric softener, without colour fixer. Can this work? Rest assured: it works! Our homemade detergents make the laundry spotlessly clean, keep the colours bright and make the laundry fluffy and soft. And we can still have the fresh scent of the laundry, knowing exactly where it comes from and that it does not irritate our skin.

The advertising industry claims almost magical powers for their detergent products. Whoever buys and uses their products, they say, can solve any laundry problem. But there is in fact nothing magical about the cleaning power of these products: they simply rely on the concentrated use of bleaching agents and optical brighteners. Many of the so-called super detergents on offer differ only in the proportion of

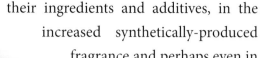

their ingredients and additives, in the increased synthetically-produced fragrance and perhaps even in the added artificial colour of the powder or liquid.

Homemade detergents contain only the additives that *we* choose. We can pick from a variety of natural substances that neither trigger allergies nor turn wastewater into a chemical cocktail. The residues that remain in the garments after each wash do not irritate our skin, nor do they penetrate through the skin into our body, where in the worst case they affect the immune system and hormone balance. Special recipes have been included for those with *very* hard water (*see* pages 121, 122).

Before we start with the production of our detergents, here are a few tips and tricks that will make the actual washing process simpler and often also reduce the amount of detergents we use.

LAUNDRY MUST BE SORTED before washing. It makes no sense to stuff a pillowcase into the washing machine together with a pair of work trousers, just in order to make it full. First the laundry should be sorted by colour. Obviously you should never wash white laundry with coloured laundry. But you also shouldn't wash lingerie in intense, bright colours together with pastel shades or even black. And finally, robust fabrics should be separated from fine, sensitive fabrics. If these factors are taken into account, the washing process can be adapted precisely to the requirements of the laundry, which in the long run avoids wasting time, energy, cost and often the annoyance of a garment that has become unwearable after a wash.

TOWELS AND BED LINEN need a higher temperature during washing. They tend to form lint and fluff so they should therefore be washed separately from all other laundry.

TROUSERS, JACKETS, SHIRTS AND BLOUSES should always be checked to see if pockets are empty before putting the item into the washing machine. Anyone who has experienced what a paper tissue forgotten in a trouser pocket can do, will agree.

THE CORRECT WATER TEMPERATURE for washing can be found on the sewn-in labels of (almost) all textiles. Stick to them, to prevent shrinking garments, or in many cases wash at a lower temperature. If textiles are recommended for washing at temperatures of 40°C, for example, they will be just as clean at 30°C. Calculated over the year, this will make a difference in electricity consumption.

WASHING IN COLD WATER has its advantages. With a cold wash, the garments do not shrink, and textiles with rich colours do not fade, nor pass their colour on to other items in the washing machine. But only slightly soiled laundry and sensitive textiles should *always* be washed cold. Washing with warm water (up to 40 °C) has the advantage that the laundry hardly creases. Machine washable wool, synthetic fabrics and black clothes should be washed warm.

HEAVILY SOILED CLOTHING without synthetic fibres such as towels, bed linen and white linen, but under no circumstances made of pure wool, can tolerate washing in hot water (60 to 90°C). The boiling of bed linen should be reserved only for cases of disease.

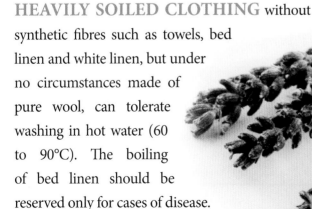

Although TENNIS BALLS in the laundry sound strange, they have one remarkable advantage: they mimic the 'pounding' of laundry which used to take place in pre-washing machine times. The pounding makes it easier to remove the dirt from the fabric. The tennis balls in the laundry knock the fabric evenly and regularly through their movement in the washing drum, which loosens dirt deep in the fabric – and that saves detergent. It goes without saying that the tennis balls should not have been on a tennis court or in a dog's mouth before they are used in the washing machine. And of course, instead of tennis balls, you can also use special washing balls, made for exactly this purpose. With wool and very sensitive laundry items, however, the use of washing balls or tennis balls should be avoided, as wool can become felted from the heavy stress.

White wine VINEGAR or fruit vinegar should always be within easy reach of the washing machine! Vinegar makes the fabric soft and fluffy, making it an effective fabric softener. It also dissolves uric acid – useful to all who need to wash baby clothes. It also removes detergent residues from the fabric. If you put laundry in the tumble dryer for drying, a final rinse with vinegar prevents the laundry from sticking together by charging it with static electricity in the tumble dryer.

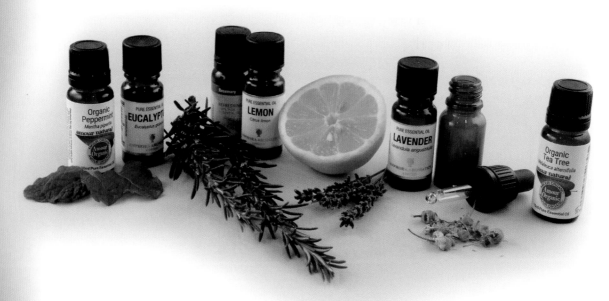

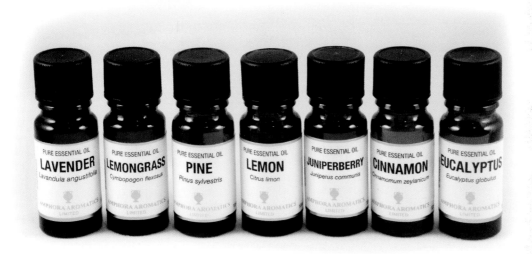

HARD WATER is a problem in many areas because it reduces the effectiveness of detergents and causes calcification of the washing machine. If the water hardness is not too high, the bicarbonate of soda in most of our homemade detergents is sufficient to render the mineral substances present in the water largely harmless. If the water is very hard, you should also sprinkle bicarbonate of soda, violet root powder or zeolite powder over the laundry as a water softener. *See also* pp 121, 122.

You will achieve FRAGRANT LAUNDRY by adding essential oils to your homemade detergents. Simply add a few drops of your favourite oil to the detergent, whether it is a powder or a liquid. You can also put the essential oil in the fabric softener if you use one. The essential oils not only give the laundry a fresh, pleasant scent, they also increase the washing power of the detergent through their grease-dissolving action. If you sometimes suffer from fungal infections, you can even use essential oil in the detergent to prevent them. Simply add about ten drops of essential tea tree oil to each wash. And if someone is fighting a persistent cold, you can do the same with essential eucalyptus oil and thus make a contribution to recovery.

If you use BICARBONATE OF SODA as a water softener, it can be ready-mixed with your chosen essential oil. Add about 20 drops of the selected essential oil to half a kilogram of bicarbonate of soda and mix the two ingredients well. Even those who use vinegar as a fabric softener can add the essential oil to it. In this case, add three to five drops of essential oil to a cup of vinegar – the necessary amount for one wash.

If you want to use essential oils not only for their cleansing power and fragrance, but also for your WELL-BEING, you can choose from a range of oils. They release their effect through the molecules, which remain suspended between the fibres of the fabric even after a piece of laundry has dried, and are only released from the fabric by the movement of the fibres when they are worn.

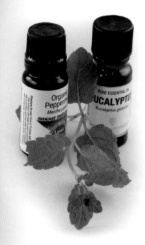

Eucalyptus oil and peppermint oil
work very well against colds and problems
with the sinuses.

Camomile oil and lavender oil
have a calming and relaxing effect.

Rosemary oil and lemon oil
have a stimulating effect and promote
concentration.

Tea tree oil
has an antibacterial effect and kills fungi,
germs and spores.

Almost any essential oil is suitable for
adding a special, characteristic fragrance to
lingerie, whichever is your
personal favourite.

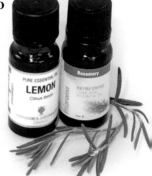

STAIN REMOVERS

The easiest way to remove stains is to treat them with the appropriate stain remover as soon as possible. Use only cold water! Warm water can cause fruit stains and stains of liquids containing sugar to spread and settle into the fabric. If you try to remove the stains before washing the garment, nothing is lost. Washing which has dried and stubborn stains should be soaked for at least half an hour before washing. This also applies to other heavily soiled laundry.

In both cases – stains and heavy soiling – one can use a simple pre-treatment spray:

100ml surgical spirit
100ml white vinegar

These two ingredients are mixed and filled into a spray bottle. Spray the stains on the spread-out garments with the mixture. Leave to soak in for about a quarter of an hour, then wash as usual. In the case of sensitive textiles, the spray should be tested on a hidden part of the garment before application to the stain. In technical jargon, this is referred to as a 'hem sample', since any changes to the garment won't be seen if there is any damage done, especially in terms of colour.

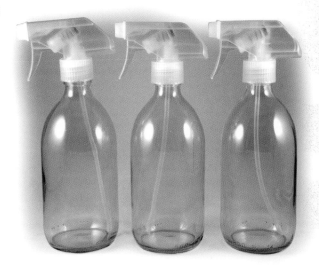

Traces of deodorant stains are particularly stubborn, especially on blouses and T-shirts where they can leave unattractive marks under the armpits, and which cannot be removed by a normal cycle in the washing machine. A special pre-treatment with washing soda is recommended.

Dissolve three tablespoons of washing soda in half a litre of hot water, place the garment in a second plastic tub and pour the soda solution over it so that the stained areas are well covered. Then sprinkle two tablespoons of washing soda directly on the stains. Allow to soak in a little, then rub the stained areas against each other. It begins to smear and foam easily, and this is the sign that the stains are loosening. Then rinse briefly and wash the item in the washing machine as usual.

The following pre-wash products for stained laundry usually contain vinegar. However, some colours, especially synthetic textiles, can fade due to vinegar. If in doubt, the pre-treatment agent should be tested on a hidden part of the garment. If there are no signs of fading or colour change, it can be used with confidence.

PRE-WASH SOAKING AGENT FOR STAINED LAUNDRY

150ml white vinegar
30g salt
5 drops essential tea tree oil

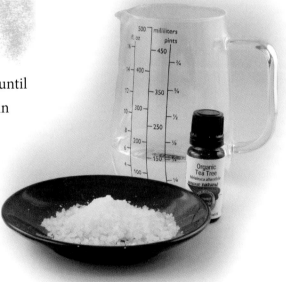

The salt is stirred in the vinegar until completely dissolved. Then stir in the essential tea tree oil. Place the stained garments in a plastic tub and add enough warm (not hot!) water over them to cover fully, then add the soaking agent. The garments should be soaked in this solution for at least one hour.

Then you can machine wash them as usual and even stubborn stains should disappear.

EASY SWEAT REMOVER LIQUID

100ml white vinegar
15g bicarbonate of soda
5 drops essential eucalyptus or citrus oil

The bicarbonate of soda is mixed thoroughly in the vinegar. Then add the essential oil, stir well again and pour the solution over the sweat stains. With a soft cloth or with the fingertips, rub the solution well into the fabric. Then machine wash the garment as usual.

SOAKING AGENT FOR SWEAT STAINS

50ml lemon juice
150ml white vinegar
5 drops essential tea tree oil

The juice of a lemon is poured through a coffee filter to remove even the finest pulp to avoid any being trapped in the fabric of the garment during the washing process. Then mix the lemon juice with the vinegar and the tea tree oil.

Soak the sweat-stained garment in a plastic tub or bathtub in warm water and then pour the soaking agent over it. The soaking time should not be less than one hour: two hours are recommended. Then wash as usual in the washing machine.

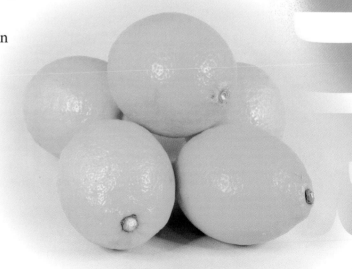

ALL-ROUND STAIN SPRAY

100ml liquid soap
30g bicarbonate of soda
50ml glycerine
150ml water
10 drops essential tea tree oil

All ingredients are well mixed and filled into a spray bottle. This stain remover is very useful for fresh food and drink stains. The stain is sprayed extensively with it, allowed to act briefly and the stain should then be able to be washed out easily with lukewarm water.

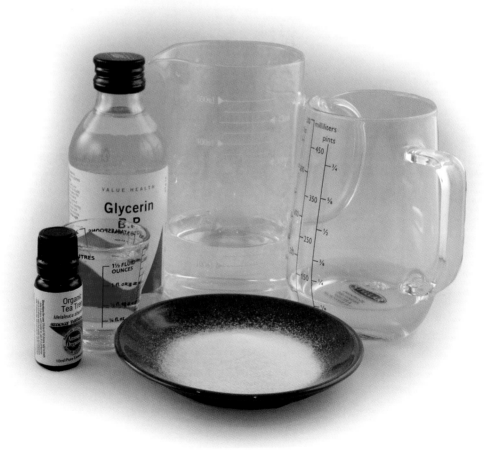

ALL-ROUND STAIN SPRAY

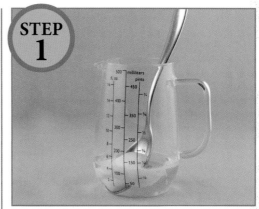

STEP 1

Stir the soda into the liquid soap.

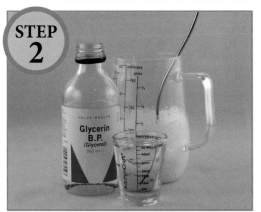

STEP 2

Stir in the glycerine.

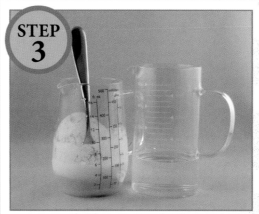

STEP 3

Add water and mix.

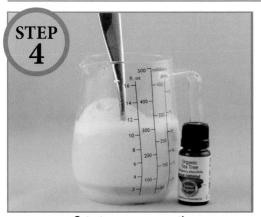

STEP 4

Stir in tea tree oil.

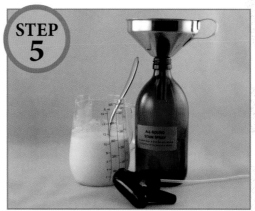

STEP 5

Store in a spray bottle.

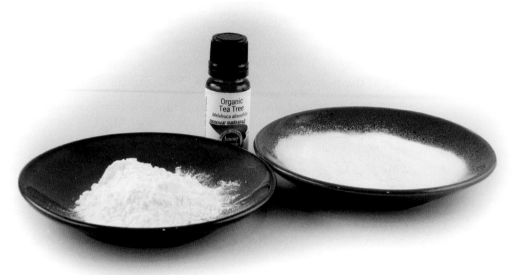

STAIN-KILLER PASTE

20g cream of tartar
50g bicarbonate of soda
5 drops essential tea tree oil
some warm water

Mix the cream of tartar, bicarbonate of soda and essential tea tree oil well together and stir by the spoonful with warm water until a smooth paste is obtained. This paste is applied to the stain caused by food or drink (even stains from gravy or coffee will be demolished by this paste!) and allowed to dry completely. Then you can wash the garment in the washing machine. The stain will have vanished.

21 COMMON STAINS

Many of the stains that plague our clothing are real individualists. You can't deal with them en bloc. These include the truly stubborn spots such as those from berries, red wine, blood or ink. And because they are all so different, specific stains and the appropriate means and methods for removing them are listed below. You may have to use one or two different remedies a couple of times before the stain completely disappears. In between stain-removing sessions, you should not put the garment in the tumble dryer, but let it dry in the air. The tumble dryer can act as a real stain fixer!

BABY FOOD usually contains soy protein and this causes stubborn stains. Even if these are washed out immediately, an outline stain may still be seen after a machine wash. The remedy is a mixture of vinegar and finely crushed garlic or garlic juice. Rub the stain vigorously with this, and the soy protein will be removed from the fabric.

BERRY STAINS usually have a nice red or blue colour, but they are undesirable as a design element on your shirt-front. So before the berry stain has dried, it should be rubbed with a slice of lemon and it should vanish. Once the berry stains have dried, things get more complicated. However, the following method of stain removal has proved its worth: rub the stain with glycerine and let it work for a good half hour before washing it out and allowing the garment to dry in the air.

If you can still see the stain, mix together the following:

2 tablespoons cornflour
1 tablespoon glycerine
5 drops of essential eucalyptus oil.

Stirring constantly, add just enough water by the spoonful to produce a smooth paste. Apply this thickly to the stain and place the garment in the sun to dry. Then brush the dried paste out. If the stain is *very* stubborn, it may be necessary to repeat this procedure several times. But in the end you will be the victor, not the stain!

THE PENCIL is one of the most useful devices invented by mankind. However, if it leaves traces on the sleeves or cuffs of shirts or blouses, these usually do not disappear during normal machine washing. But there is a very simple trick: Take an eraser (a rubber) to it before washing, and erase the pencil marks!

BLOOD STAINS stick stubbornly in fabric, but can be removed with a certain amount of patience. It is best to soak the bloodstained garment immediately in a solution of cold water and detergent and leave it in there for several hours. At temperatures above 40 °C, blood components coagulate and become set in the material. But after a good soak in cold water, the blood stain can be rubbed out with a soft cloth. If it cannot be completely removed in this way, it can be dealt with using hydrogen peroxide. Rub with a cloth generously moistened in hydrogen peroxide until the stain is gone.... and if all this fails, cut your losses and rip the garment into shoe-cleaning rags!

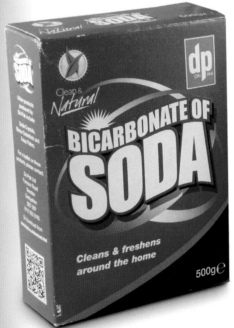

BUTTER OR MARGARINE can leave greasy stains that cannot be completely removed by normal machine washing. A paste consisting of a tablespoon of bicarbonate of soda, three drops of essential citrus oil and a little water applied to the stain and dried for about an hour solves this problem and leaves no trace of the stain.

FAT AND OIL stains are particularly problematic in that the fat is quickly distributed in the fibres of the fabric and only part of it remains on the surface of the fabric. The sooner you start to remove the grease stain, the easier it will be. Mix one tablespoon each of bicarbonate of soda, salt and cornflour, sprinkle this mixture on the stain and let it work for at least half an hour. Then wipe it away and soak the part of the garment with the stain in diluted vinegar with a few drops of essential citrus oil. After about an hour the grease stain should be completely removed and the garment can be machine washed as usual.

GRASS STAINS are often part of a happy memory, but still have to be removed from the garment. Soak the area with the grass stain in vinegar, let it work for about half an hour, then spread a paste of bicarbonate of soda and water on the stain. Let it dry and then put it in the washing machine.

COFFEE AND TEA cause dark stains, which should be treated as soon as possible. The quickest way to do this is to pour milk over the fresh stain, rub a little so that the milk can dissolve the liquid that has penetrated deeper into the fabric, then dab with a soft cloth. This process may have to be repeated several times. Then warm water can be used to remove the remains of milk and milk fat from the fabric. The tannins in tea and coffee are used as natural dyes, which makes their removal considerably more difficult after some time.

The best way to remove a dried coffee or tea stain is to soak the stained part of the garment in a solution of water and soda powder for several hours before washing.

CHEWING GUM stains usually arise because you've sat on a discarded piece. The best way to get rid of chewing gum is to put the affected piece of clothing in a plastic bag and put it in the freezer for at least half an hour. The chewing gum residue and stain can then be easily removed. In the event that traces are still visible, they can be soaked in vinegar before machine washing.

CANDLE WAX can be removed from textiles in a similar way to chewing gum. Because wax usually drips on the sleeves of shirts or blouses, you don't necessarily have to freeze the whole item. It is often enough to place an ice cube on the wax stain and let it harden. Then you carefully scrape off the hard wax. If there are any traces remaining in the fabric, place this part of the garment between two paper tissues or pieces of paper kitchen roll and iron carefully with a warm iron (temperature setting for silk) until the papers have completely absorbed the liquid wax.

LIPSTICK STAINS can be rubbed with white toothpaste regardless of their colour and then carefully dabbed with a soft damp cloth. If traces are still visible, you can either repeat the procedure or dab the spot several times with essential eucalyptus oil. After the subsequent machine washing, the stain should no longer be visible.

MOULD STAINS are a problem that can often arise, for example, in the summer after a long day by the swimming pool. You put the towels in a bag and forget them. These are the ideal conditions for the development of mould. But the stains are relatively easy to get rid of:

1 cup vinegar
1 tablespoon salt
5 drops essential tea tree oil

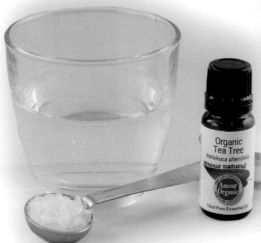

Stir together the above ingredients and soak the mildew stains in it. Then hand over the towels to the washing machine!

NAIL POLISH sometimes leaves stains, no matter how careful you are. It might seem to make most sense to immediately remove nail polish with nail polish remover. However, nail polish removers usually contain acetone as a solvent, and this solvent can also attack or dissolve synthetic fibres. You should therefore test whether the garment tolerates this treatment on a hidden part of the garment such as the hem. If not, you can try cleaning with surgical spirit.

RUST STAINS are among the most persistent. If the fabric of the garment tolerates boiling water, you can get rid of them with a little effort. First make a liquid paste from lemon juice and salt and spread it on the rust stain. Allow to work for about a quarter of an hour, then rinse well with very hot to boiling water.

An old household remedy is suitable for rust-stained textiles that do not tolerate hot water. However, it is linked to the season of fresh asparagus. Take two fresh sticks of asparagus and boil them in about half a litre of water. After cooling down, you can soak the rust-stained garment in it for several hours. It is then washed in the machine as usual.

SALAD DRESSING can cause quite resistant stains. A universal remedy, however, is a solution consisting of

100ml vinegar
50ml lemon juice
10 drops of essential citrus oil.
Soak the stained part of the garment in this solution for about an hour and then wash it normally in the machine.

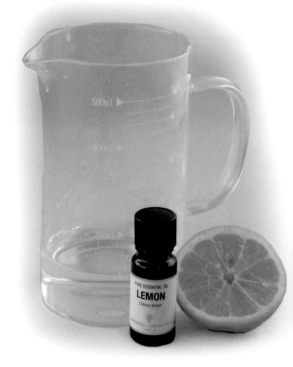

CHOCOLATE STAINS require a paste of bicarbonate of soda and water. You apply it to the stain, let it dry and then machine wash the garment as normal. The chocolate stain should completely disappear.

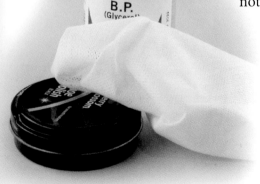

SHOE POLISH leaves stains that should never be treated with water. It makes them worse! It is best to put glycerine on a soft cloth and rub the stain carefully with it. The garment can then be machine washed.

MUSTARD STAINS are bright yellow, but not in a good way on your clothes. They can be removed from the material by spraying them with glycerine and letting it work for about an hour. Then carefully rub soda powder into the stain and put the garment into the washing machine.

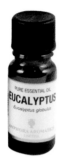

INK STAINS have ruined many a white shirt. Essential eucalyptus oil is a good solvent for ink – also for waterproof ink. Place a cloth under the spot of the garment with the stain and drizzle the eucalyptus oil on it. The ink then seeps through the fabric into the cloth underneath. Take care that no part of the garment gets under the cloth and gets some of the dissolved ink.

If after this treatment you can still see the remains of the stain, you can soak the garment in a mixture of equal parts of vinegar and milk before washing.

URINE STAINS disappear if the garment or its stained part is soaked in a mixture of vinegar, warm water (equal parts) and ten drops of essential lavender oil before washing.

WINE STAINS should be rinsed out immediately with water. If edges are still visible, you can rub the spot with a slice of lemon. Then put the garment in the washing machine and wash as usual.

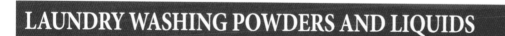

LAUNDRY WASHING POWDERS AND LIQUIDS

Industrially-produced detergents have been around for less than 100 years. Before that, it was customary to make your own detergents. Of course, washing laundry used to be a much more strenuous activity than it is today, when we can simply stuff the laundry into the washing machine and set off the appropriate washing programme. However, with the simplification of washing, the demand for clean clothes has increased significantly. Luckily, our homemade detergents

with health-friendly ingredients are just as good as the industrial products with their often unsound ingredients and additives.

The detergents of our ancestors were based either on soaps or, before that, on ash. They used wood-burner ash, which was mixed with water, filtered and then used as a kind of liquid detergent. The potash contained in the ash is a powerful fat solvent. Not much more is known about the ancient recipe of this detergent. Because it is often difficult today to get sufficient amounts of ash, this book will deal with soap-based detergents.

Natural soap without perfumes and other additives in liquid or solid form or as soap flakes is suitable for the production of detergents. Whether curd soap or Castile soap made from coconut or olive oil, one can produce effective washing powders and liquid detergents from it. Soap is particularly suitable for laundry washing because it does not, like the surfactants in commercial detergents, completely de-grease the fibres. It de-greases adequately, but has a slight moisturising effect. This makes the fabrics soft and makes the use of conventional fabric softeners largely superfluous.

You can add to the detergent the fragrance you like best for your laundry, in the form of essential oils. The essential oils not only provide the laundry with fragrance,

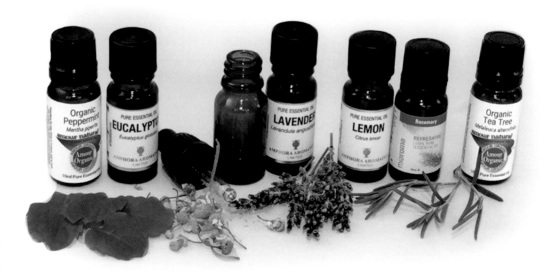

they also increase the washing power of your homemade detergent. The essential oils of spruce, cedar, pine, eucalyptus, lavender, lemon, orange, lime, peppermint, geranium, rosemary and tea tree are particularly suitable for clothes washing. You can use them individually or combine them to create your own personal fragrance.

LAUNDRY LIQUID FROM CURD SOAP

100g grated curd soap, or soap flakes
150ml boiling water
20g bicarbonate of soda
10 drops of essential oil of your choice

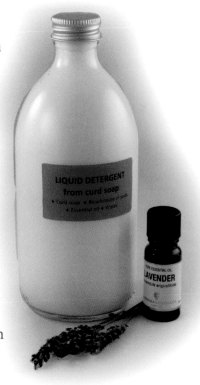

Place the grated curd soap or soap flakes in a large pan or bowl, pour the boiling water over and stir until the soap has completely dissolved. Then stir in the soda powder until completely dissolved, and finally add the essential oil. Then pour the detergent into a suitable storage bottle.

As with all liquid detergents, pour into the correct compartment of the washing machine. You can use considerably less than the maximum mark, unless you have particularly heavily soiled laundry. And even in this case, no need to use an excessive amount.

LAUNDRY LIQUID FROM CURD SOAP

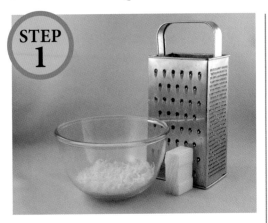

STEP 1

Grate the curd soap into flakes.

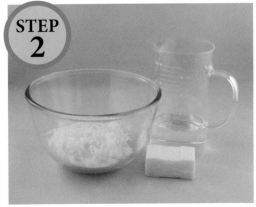

STEP 2

Pour boiling water over...

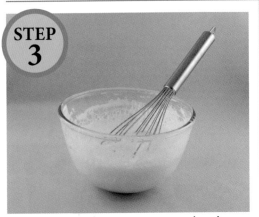

STEP 3

Stir until the soap is completely dissolved.

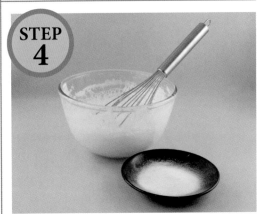

STEP 4

Stir in the soda.

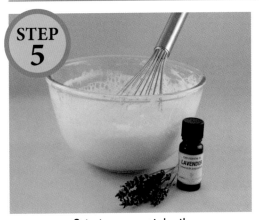

STEP 5

Stir in essential oil.

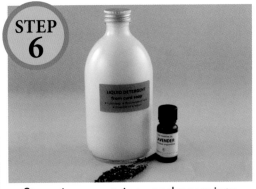

STEP 6

Store in a container and pour into the detergent compartment of the washing machine.

LAUNDRY LIQUID FROM LIQUID SOAP //

150ml liquid curd soap or Castile liquid soap
100ml hot water
30g bicarbonate of soda
20g washing soda
10 drops of essential oil of your choice

Mix the liquid soap with the hot water until it is completely dissolved. Stir in the bicarbonate of soda and washing soda and finally the essential oil, then pour the finished detergent into a storage bottle. It is used exactly as you would other liquid detergents.

LIQUID DETERGENT WITH GLYCERINE //////////////////////////

500ml liquid curd soap or
        Castile liquid soap
20ml glycerine
20 drops of essential oil of your choice

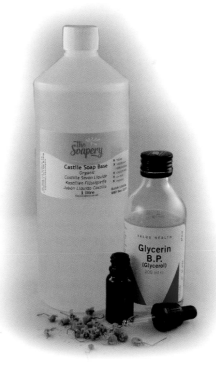

Glycerine and essential oil are mixed into the liquid soap and poured into a suitable, airtight bottle. For one wash cycle you need to fill the appropriate compartment of the washing machine, having shaken the bottle well. The essential oils tend to settle at the bottom of the bottle.

SPECIAL DETERGENT FOR WHITE COTTON WASHING

150ml white vinegar
100ml water
30g bicarbonate of soda
10g citric acid
10 drops essential citrus oil

The vinegar is mixed with the water, then the bicarbonate of soda and citric acid are added and stirred until these powdery ingredients are completely dissolved. Then stir in the essential citrus oil and pour the detergent into a suitable storage bottle.

MILD DETERGENT FOR KNITWEAR AND LINGERIE

250ml liquid soap (liquid curd soap or Castile liquid soap)
30g dried rosemary
250ml boiling water

Rosemary has always been regarded as a proven product for the care of very sensitive knitwear and fine lingerie. The only exceptions for this detergent are knitwear made of pure wool, and textiles made of silk or satin – do not use this rosemary detergent on these materials.

The dried rosemary is finely ground in a mortar so that its essential oils can permeate the water. Tip the ground rosemary into a suitable pan or bowl with the boiling water. Cover and leave to stand for about 20 minutes. Strain and stir with the liquid soap until completely dissolved. Then fill into a bottle that can be closed tightly.

Approximately 150ml of this detergent is required for one wash. Washing is carried out cold or at a maximum temperature of 30°C and in the gentle cycle of the machine.

LIQUID DETERGENT FOR COLOURED FABRICS

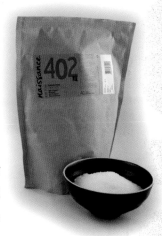

200ml liquid curd soap or Castile liquid soap
50g washing soda
100g Epsom salts (magnesium sulphate)
300ml water
15 drops of essential oil of your choice

Washing soda and Epsom salts are stirred into the water until they are completely dissolved. Then stir in the liquid soap and finally the essential oil and pour the detergent into a suitable, tightly-sealed bottle.

This detergent is particularly suitable for textiles with rich, bright colours. For one wash you need about 150-200ml.

LAUNDRY WASHING POWDER

SOAP-BASED WASHING POWDER

50g washing soda
50g bicarbonate of soda
50g soap flakes
10 drops of essential oil of your choice

Washing soda and soda powder are well mixed and drizzled with the essential oil. Then you mix in the soap flakes and stir the whole lot again well. This washing powder can also be produced in larger quantities and filled into an airtight plastic container (especially suitable: the half or 1 litre plastic ice-cream container as soon as they are emptied!)

Use this washing powder in the appropriate compartment of the washing machine. Or you can also sprinkle it directly over the laundry in the machine. It is ideally suited for washing temperatures from 40 to 90 °C.

WASHING POWDER

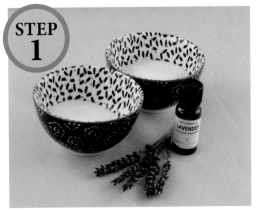

Mix soda and bicarbonate of soda with the essential oil.

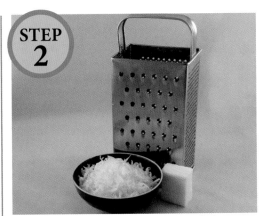

Grate the curd soap into flakes.

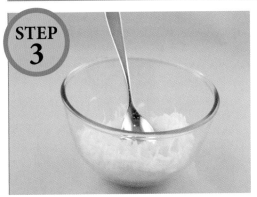

Mix the soap flakes with the mixture of soda, bicarbonate of soda and essential oil.

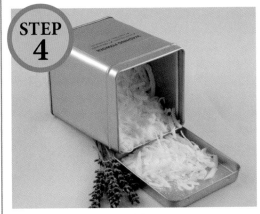

Fill into suitable container.

FRAGRANT WASHING POWDER /////////

200g soap flakes
200g washing soda
200g bicarbonate of soda
20 drops essential citrus oil
20 drops essential lavender oil
20 drops essential orange oil

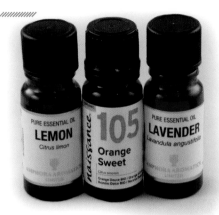

Washing soda and bicarbonate of soda are mixed well together, then the essential oils are added drop by drop, stirring constantly. Lastly, mix in the soap flakes.

This fragrant washing powder should be stored in an airtight plastic container.

SPECIAL WASHING POWDER FOR HARD WATER /////////////////////////

200g washing soda
100g bicarbonate of soda
100g soap flakes or grated curd soap

.... and the corresponding hard water fabric softener:

250ml white vinegar
10 drops essential oil of your choice

This special hard water detergent contains soap in the powder and it contains vinegar in the fabric softener – two ingredients that must *always* be separated from each other. For the washing powder, put the washing soda, bicarbonate of soda and soap flakes in a suitable bowl or pan and mix the ingredients well. Separately, mix the vinegar with the essential oil in a bottle by shaking it well. The washing powder is placed in the appropriate compartment of the washing machine or is spread directly over the laundry in the washing drum. You need about half a small cup of this powder per wash. Use the softener compartment of the washing machine for the conditioner.

POWDER FOR WATER SOFTENING

100g washing soda
100g salt
100g zeolite powder

With very hard water it can be necessary or at least helpful to use a special agent for water softening. This uses the properties of zeolite powder, a natural mineral that is also used for clarifying aquariums and ponds. The zeolite powder is mixed with washing soda and salt and sprinkled in a small amount – about half a cup per wash – directly over the laundry in the drum of the washing machine.

MILD BLEACHING AGENT

200ml water
50ml liquid soap
50g washing soda
10 drops essential citrus oil

Stir the washing soda, dissolve completely in the water then mix with the liquid soap and essential citrus oil. This bleaching agent is suitable for hand-washing white shirts and blouses, for pre-washing white laundry with stains, but also for machine washing white textiles.

BLEACH WITH LEMON

100ml lemon juice
100g bicarbonate of soda
150ml water

Dissolve the soda powder completely in the water by stirring and then mix with the lemon juice. In order to remove any remains of fruit flesh, you should strain the lemon juice through a coffee filter. Because the freshly squeezed lemon juice does not have a very long shelf life, no large quantities of this bleaching agent should be produced in advance. The ingredients listed above are sufficient for one wash.

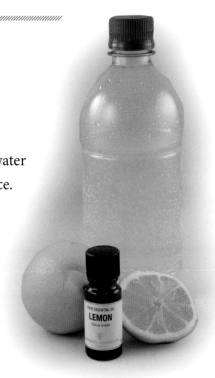

FABRIC SOFTENERS

Vinegar is unbeatable as a fabric softener. It is natural, guaranteed free of harmful additives and has the advantage of removing all detergent residues from the fabric during the rinse cycle. It is also possible to add any desired fragrance – flowery, woody, herbal – in the form of essential oils.

With white laundry, vinegar is unproblematic as a fabric softener, concerning the quantity used. However, with coloured laundry one should dose very sparingly, because vinegar can lead to colour running. This applies especially to textiles made of viscose.

LAUNDRY

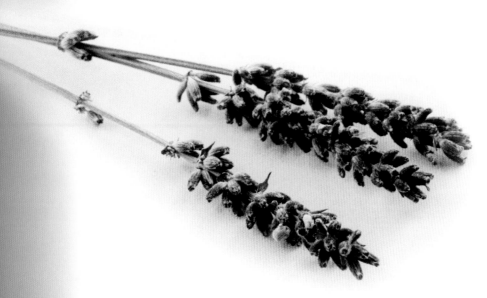

LAVENDER FABRIC SOFTENER

750ml white vinegar
25 drops essential lavender oil

If you pour the essential lavender oil directly into the vinegar bottle and shake it well, you always have a fabric softener to hand. It is also very effective. Before use, shake the bottle thoroughly so that the essential oil is evenly distributed in the vinegar and does not settle on the bottom.

PEPPERMINT FABRIC SOFTENER

750ml white wine vinegar
15 drops essential peppermint oil

Add the essential peppermint oil drop by drop to the vinegar bottle and shake it thoroughly so that the essential oil is evenly distributed in the vinegar. Use in the fabric softener compartment of the washing machine.

ORANGE FABRIC SOFTENER

50g bicarbonate of soda
250ml water
750ml white vinegar
25 drops essential orange oil

The bicarbonate of soda powder is completely dissolved in the water by stirring, then the vinegar added and stirred again well. Finally, the essential orange oil is stirred in and the finished fabric softener is filled into a suitable bottle. Of course, you could use the original vinegar bottle.

Used in the fabric softener compartment of the washing machine, it gives the laundry a fresh, fruity scent and prevents clothes clinging together in the tumble dryer due to static electricity.

LEMON FABRIC SOFTENER

750ml white vinegar
100ml water
50g bicarbonate of soda
15 drops essential citrus oil

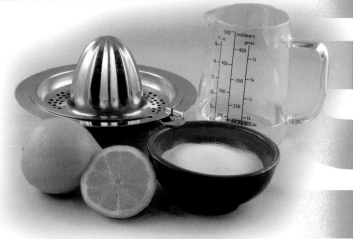

The bicarbonate of soda is stirred in the water until completely dissolved and poured into the vinegar. Stir well again, then stir in the essential citrus oil. The best container to use is the vinegar bottle. Use in the fabric softener compartment of the washing machine, and your laundry smells delicately of fresh lemon!

FABRIC SOFTENER WITH HERB VINEGAR

Those who can't use essential oils, whether because of allergies, pregnancy or small children, can introduce the scent and power of the herbs directly into the vinegar. You just make concentrated herb vinegar!

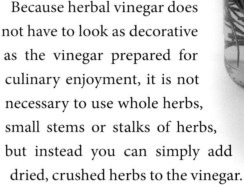

Because herbal vinegar does not have to look as decorative as the vinegar prepared for culinary enjoyment, it is not necessary to use whole herbs, small stems or stalks of herbs, but instead you can simply add dried, crushed herbs to the vinegar.

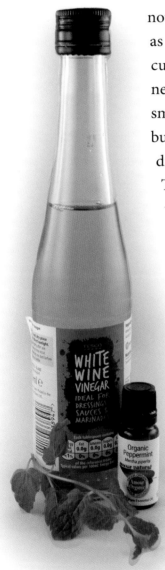

This has the advantage that the vinegar can absorb the active ingredients of the herbs much faster. It is usually sufficient to leave the dried herbs in the vinegar for a week. If you are using whole fresh herbs, it takes three to four weeks.

We therefore use dried herbs for the production of fabric softener herb vinegar. Rosemary, peppermint, lemon balm and lavender are the most common herbs. However, you can try other fragrant herbs.

Put three to four heaped tablespoons of the dried and chopped herbs into a large glass jar and pour the vinegar over it. Close the jar tightly, shake thoroughly and place in a warm, but not sunny place. The bottle should be shaken thoroughly at least once a day, so that fresh vinegar and herbs are always in direct contact. After a week, strain the mixture through a fine sieve and pour it into a suitable bottle. You now have a fabric softener with additional herbal power that can be poured into the fabric softener compartment of the washing machine.

LAUNDRY PERFUME

This was once an essential prerequisite in grand households. There were no fabric softeners, and homemade detergents with the scent of essential oils were not yet common, so the laundry got its fresh scent in the way I'm about to explain. You can easily make your own laundry perfume and spray it sparingly on the laundry before ironing. Use 90 per cent surgical spirit, and add ten drops of essential oil of your choice to 100ml of the spirit. The oil should be very light coloured or, even better, completely transparent, so that it does not leave stains on white laundry.

FRAGRANT STARCH

Starched shirt or blouse collars and cuffs have become just as rare today as starched table linen. Those who want to spoil themselves with this luxury are not dependent on the starch available on the market. You can also produce your own starch naturally and free of unwanted ingredients.

200ml water
20g cornflour
5 drops essential tea tree oil

The cornflour is stirred into the water until it has completely dissolved. Then stir in the essential tea tree oil and decant into a spray bottle. The laundry you wish to starch is sprayed sparingly then ironed as usual. Instead of tea tree oil you can also use other essential oils but they should be very pale to transparent so that they do not stain the laundry.

GREEN CLEAN YOUR HOME 127

WOOL AND SILK

Fine natural fibres such as wool and silk require particular care. Pure wool garments should only be washed by hand with liquid soap in cold water, pressing a little, but do not rub, then rinse thoroughly in cold water. Soaking and wringing damages the wool, and excessive machine washing can lead to felting. After rinsing, place the item on a dry towel and roll up in a sausage, to gently remove water from the garment. Repeat the process with a second dry towel. Finally, you need a third dry towel on which you lay the item, pull it into shape and let it dry. Woollen clothes should always be left to dry lying on a towel. They lose their shape when hung on a clothes line. Wool can bind more than twice the volume of water, and even if wool feels 'dry', there is still a lot of water stored in the fibre.

To remove a **STAIN FROM A WOOLLEN SWEATER** or jacket, moisten a cotton wool ball with white vinegar and dab the stain with it. But under no circumstances should you rub it! Let the vinegar soak in a little, then press a clean dry cloth onto the stain to transfer the vinegar to the cloth.

SILK is a product of silkworms that squeeze fine thread out of their spinning glands. The silk fibres consist of protein molecules which do not tolerate soap with a pH above ten. Silk fibres have a natural fat coating. This must be retained during washing, otherwise the silk loses its lustre and becomes dull and matt. In addition, this natural grease coating protects the silk from stains and discoloration and has the advantage that stains remain on the surface of the fabric and don't penetrate into the fibres. They can therefore be removed more easily – normal hand washing is usually sufficient. It is essential to protect silk from strong alkaline detergents and from stress in the washing machine.

For **HAND WASHING** in the sink, add at most a quarter of a cup of liquid soap to the cold or lukewarm water and mix with your hand. In this dilution the pH value of the washing solution won't damage the silk. Then the silk garment is placed in the water and submerged several times. **Do not leave to soak**. Then rinse the items thoroughly with cold or lukewarm water. Wringing or twisting should be avoided, otherwise the silk will crease. After rinsing, place the garment on a dry towel and use your flat hands to squeeze the remaining water out of the fabric. To dry, you can hang up the silk garment, but not with clothes pegs – instead, use a wide coat hanger, preferably made of wood or plastic, not metal.

White silk garments must be washed particularly carefully. Even so, with increasing age the silk can turn a little yellow. These signs of aging can be counteracted easily. Wash the piece as described above, but omit the soap, using

50ml white vinegar
30ml hydrogen peroxide
5 drops essential tea tree oil

in the washing water. Mix these three ingredients in a glass bowl with about half a litre of lukewarm water and pour them into the washbasin filled with water. Mix by hand and submerge the silk garment several times. Then rinse and dry as described above.

By the way: you only iron things made of silk inside out, otherwise they lose their 'silky' shine!

DRYING

Today, laundry is often no longer dried by the wind, but is put in the tumble dryer after washing. Tumble drying is more gentle on the laundry if tumble dryer sheets are used. You put one or two of them in the drum and they have the added advantage that you can scent the laundry during drying. You can easily make them yourself, using your individual favourite fragrance. Use cellulose cloths, which you can buy cheaply on rolls then cut them down to the right size – about 20 x 20 centimetres.

FRAGRANT TUMBLE DRYER SHEETS

25 cellulose wipes, cut to size
200ml water
20ml of surgical spirit
5g glycerine
25 drops of essential oil of your choice

The cellulose wipes are placed in an airtight sandwich box or similar. Mix the water, alcohol, glycerine and essential oil, then pour it over the wipes. When all the cloths have soaked up the mixture, any remaining liquid can be drained off and further cloths soaked with it. The amount of essential oil you use is simply a recommendation: some like a more subtle, some a more intense fragrance. You can mix different essential oils to create your own individual laundry fragrance or limit yourself to a single essential oil depending on the type of laundry. So a male-woody scent for shirts and men's underwear (cedar, patchouli), a fresh, earthy scent for outerwear (rosemary, thyme), a flowery scent for light summer dresses (geranium, orange blossom), a romantic scent for fine blouses and underwear (jasmine, ylang-ylang) or a relaxing scent for bed linen (camomile, hyssop).

IRONING

Even in times of easy-care or 'non-iron' textiles, ironing is still the best way to make a garment look clean, fresh, smart and simply beautiful. With today's generation of steam irons, this is far easier than it was in the days when you had to use a damp cloth to press your clothes. The steam iron is filled with water, ideally distilled water so that the iron will not calcify as quickly. But it doesn't have to be plain water, you can turn it into fragrant water.

FRAGRANT IRON WATER

1 litre distilled water
30ml surgical spirit
30 drops of essential oil of your choice

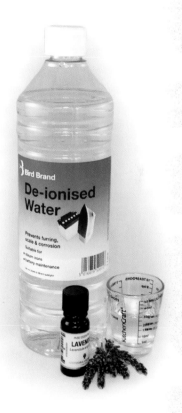

Distilled water, surgical spirit and essential oil are well mixed together and poured into a suitable, tightly-sealed bottle. The steam iron can be filled from this bottle as required. The most common essential oils for ironing water are lavender, rose, blood orange or cedar. But the whole range of fragrances is open to you.

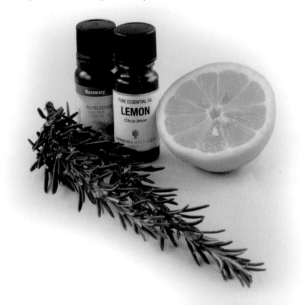

MOTHS

... love fabrics, especially garments made of natural fibres. They find their way even into the cleanest wardrobe with tightly closing doors and leave behind moth holes in your favourite clothes. For decades, people have tried to protect their clothing with the help of disgusting-smelling mothballs. As well as having an awful aroma, these old-fashioned mothballs also spread toxic naphthalene. But there are simple, natural and safe alternatives. Against moths, these homemade deterrents work just as well as poisonous mothballs.

Fabric bags of cedar wood shavings reliably protect woollens against moths. You put the cedar wood chips into a small cloth bag and put it between woollen items in a drawer.

Alternatively, you can sprinkle cellulose wipes with essential cedar oil and place them between wool clothes. The cedar scent deters moths, and they are guaranteed to lose their appetites.

Winter clothing stored in a suitcase or chest can be protected from moths with the scent of essential lavender or rosemary oil. Drip a few drops of it onto a clean tea towel, fold it up and put it between the clothes.

Winter clothes which hang open in the wardrobe during the summer become of no interest to moths if you hang dried lemon peel on the clothes rail at regular intervals. When they lose their scent after time, replace the peel.

Laundry in drawers always smells fresh and is largely safe from moths if you place a small bag of dried lavender flowers between linen in each drawer.

Drawers can also be lined with a double layer of tissue paper, the lower layer of tissue lightly rubbed with a cotton wool ball moistened with essential lavender, geranium or rosemary oil. Silk paper, also in different colours, is available in stationery and handicraft shops.

SHOES

... are mostly cleaned externally with shoe polish. However, bacteria and germs accumulate inside them, which over time causes the well-known sweaty smell. This can be avoided by spraying the insides with shoe spray. You mix

100ml water
20ml surgical spirit
30 drops essential tea tree oil

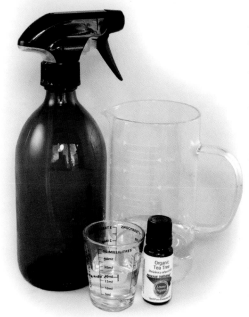

Put this mixture in a spray bottle. The spirit and tea tree oil kills off germs and bacteria and prevents the musty smell from developing in the first place.

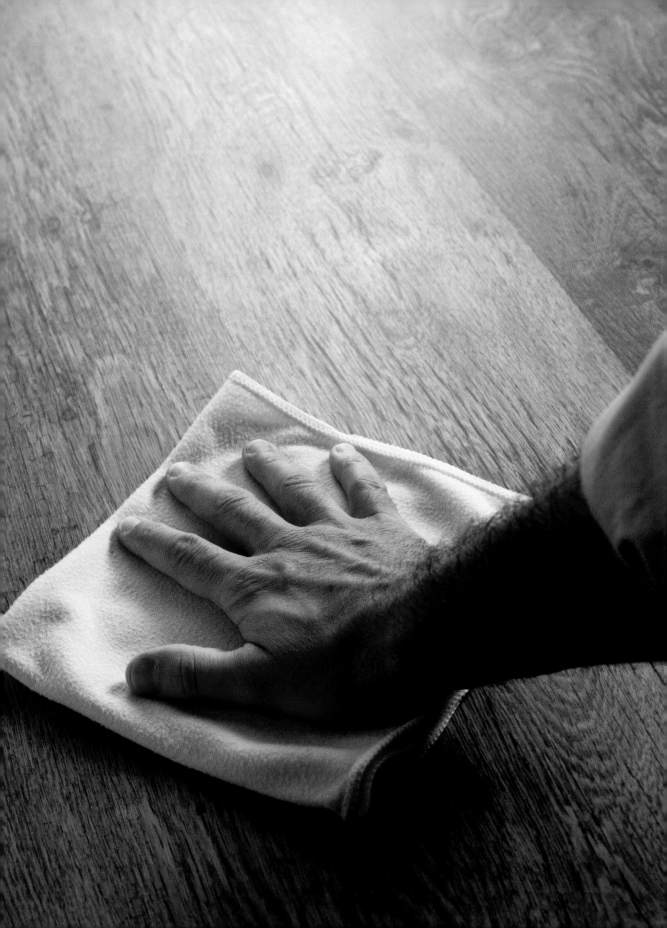

CHAPTER SEVEN

WOODEN FLOORS AND FURNITURE

WOOD IS THE MOST POPULAR MATERIAL IN OUR LIVING ENVIRONMENT AND IT NEEDS A CERTAIN AMOUNT OF CARE TO RETAIN ITS BEAUTY

Wood is a very special material. It is of course a natural material, not a manufactured one, and the very growth of the tree and its branches is reflected in the wood.

It is no wonder that we feel particularly comfortable in a living environment with a lot of wood. However, unvarnished wood surfaces take on stains. And removing them is important to keep the wood surface flawless. There are many ways and means to remove these stains. However, because different types of wood react very differently to different agents, such as essential oils, it is important to test each ingredient on a hidden part of the furniture before using it for the first time. This can be done on the underside of a table top or on the inside of a cabinet door. Only if this spot still shows no discoloration or other abnormality a few hours after application can you use the tested product without hesitation.

The care of modern living spaces is dealt with by the vacuum cleaner. For a thorough cleaning in between, for the care of upholstered furniture and carpets and for the cleaning of wooden floors and wooden furniture, however, the right cleaning and care products are needed.

BURN MARKS often occur on wooden table tops due to cigarette burns. If the stain has not burned into the surface, you can rub it off with a thin paste of cigarette ash, some linseed oil and a few drops of essential oil (tea tree for light wood, peppermint for dark wood). But if the burn mark has penetrated the wood, you will have to resort to sandpaper.

GREASE STAINS can occur on table tops and on wooden floors. In both cases, immediately place ice cubes on the grease stain so that the fat becomes hard and does not penetrate deeper into the wood fibres. A solid layer of grease forms, which can be scraped off with a blunt object such as a wooden spatula. If the grease is on varnished wood, the problem should be solved. If the wood is untreated, the outline of the grease stain may remain, in which case it can be moistened with a mixture of a little liquid soap and a few drops of essential eucalyptus oil dabbed on with a soft cloth.

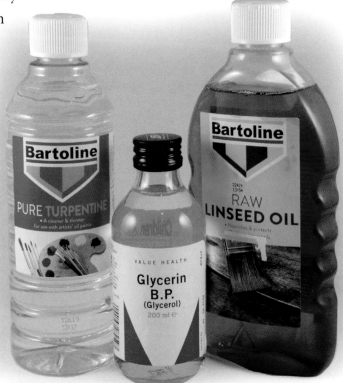

SCUFF MARKS from shoe heels often appear as black lines on wooden floors. They can usually be rubbed off with a soft cloth that has been sparingly moistened with essential cedar or eucalyptus oil.

WATER STAINS AND WATER RINGS are probably the most common stains on wooden surfaces. It doesn't even have to be leaking flower vases that cause them. Even the condensation on the outside of a cold drinking glass is enough to leave a clear water ring on the wood. To remove these stains, it is necessary to first remove the existing polish from the wood. Do this by rubbing with a cloth moistened with vinegar. Then apply linseed oil – rubbing from the outside to the inside of the water ring – and let it work for a few hours. Then polish the spot with a cloth, and the water ring or stain should not be visible.

FURNITURE CLEANER

CLEANING AGENT FOR LACQUERED WOOD

150ml water
100ml lemon juice
20ml liquid curd soap
3 drops of essential geranium or bergamot oil

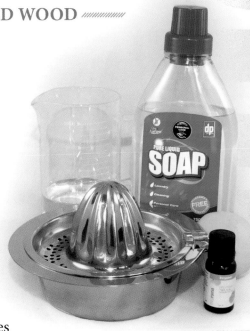

The freshly-squeezed lemon juice is poured through a coffee filter to remove the finest traces of skin and pulp. Then it is mixed with water, liquid soap and essential oil. This discreetly fragrant product can also be used to remove old, sticky or encrusted dirt from varnished wooden surfaces and gives the floor a fresh, clean appearance.

FURNITURE CLEANER WITH CEDAR SCENT

50ml liquid curd soap or Castile liquid soap
200ml water
20 drops essential cedar oil

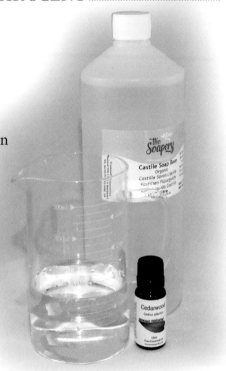

The liquid soap is mixed well with the water then
the essential cedar oil. Pour the whole thing
into a spray bottle. You now have a cleaner
for shelves, cupboard walls and doors,
chests of drawers and wooden tables,
which also removes greasy fingerprints
easily. Spray the cleaner directly onto the
surfaces and wipe them clean with a dry
cloth. As an encore you get a fresh but
unobtrusive cedar scent.

FURNITURE CLEANER WITH LEMON BALM

20g dried lemon balm
250ml boiling water
50ml lemon juice
10 drops essential citrus oil

Pour the boiling water over the dried lemon balm to cover, in a suitable bowl or
pan. Allow to steep for a good quarter of an hour, then strain. Pour the fresh lemon
juice through a coffee filter and mix with the lemon balm extract. Finally stir in the
essential citrus oil and pour the mixture into a spray bottle. If one sprays dusted
wood surfaces sparingly with this cleaner, it removes greasy dirt residues and also
ensures that the clean wood surface does not take up the dust again so quickly. It
leaves a fresh lemon scent.

WOOD FRESHENER

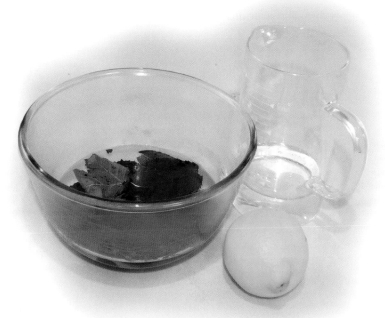

WOOD FRESHENER WITH BERRY LEAF DECOCTION

20g fresh or 10g dried raspberry or blackberry leaves
250ml boiling water
100ml white vinegar
50ml lemon juice

Pour the boiling water over the fresh or dried raspberry or blackberry leaves in a suitable pan or bowl. Allow to infuse for about 20 minutes, then strain. The freshly squeezed lemon juice is poured through a coffee filter to remove fine residues. Then mix the berry leaf decoction with vinegar and lemon juice and pour into a spray bottle.

This special cleaning agent revives old, dull wood surfaces to new freshness. Spray the cleaner on a soft cloth and wipe the surfaces with it. Wipe with a second cloth moistened with water and finally rub the surface dry with a third dry cloth.

OIL CARE

OIL CARE FOR DRY WOOD

The dry air in centrally heated rooms not only causes problems for the residents, but also for untreated or impregnated wood surfaces. The wood can become very dry and looks old. With the following remedy you can restore the freshness of this wood. It is a real 'moisture care treatment' for the wood!

100ml linseed oil
10 drops essential citrus oil

The essential citrus oil is carefully stirred into the linseed oil and poured into a suitable, airtight bottle or container. Put a little of this mixture on a clean cloth and rub the oil vigorously into the wood. It is important not to apply too much of this product to the wood surface. Oil residues attract dust, and besides, you may get oil stains on things you place on this wooden surface if you apply too much. To be on the safe side, the surface should be wiped vigorously with a clean, dry cloth about one hour after applying.

WOOD FLOOR CLEANER

Wood floors react very sensitively to moisture. If a parquet floor is often wiped wet, you can see it. If it is necessary to clean a wooden floor damp, this should be done with a moist but never dripping wet mop. A wet mop, as used for stone or tiled floors, is completely unsuitable for wood floors. The moisture can penetrate into cracks and joints and cause the wood to swell.

FLOOR CLEANER WITH CITRUS OIL

15ml liquid curd soap
500ml hot water
20 drops essential citrus oil

The liquid soap is stirred into hot water until it is completely dissolved. Then stir in the essential citrus oil and pour the whole thing into any container into which you can dip the floor cloth. You also need a bucket of clear water to rinse the wiped area again and again but first wring the cloth out firmly. This floor cleaner is intended for wooden floors and especially parquet floors, but also maintains natural stone and marble floors excellently.

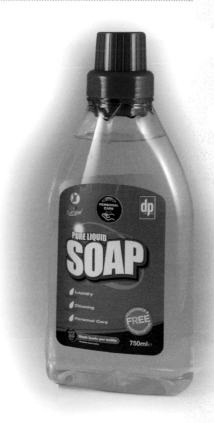

CLEANER FOR DARK WOODEN FLOORS

20g black tea
500ml boiling water
20ml liquid curd soap
20 drops essential cedar oil

Any black tea is suitable for this cleaning product. After all, it does not depend on its taste, but on the colouring and tanning agents (tannins) it contains.
Pour the boiling water over the tea, let it steep for about five minutes then strain.

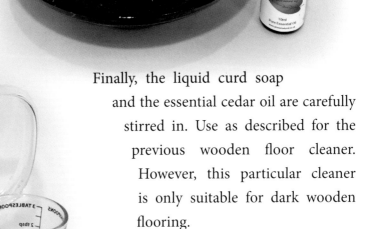

Finally, the liquid curd soap and the essential cedar oil are carefully stirred in. Use as described for the previous wooden floor cleaner. However, this particular cleaner is only suitable for dark wooden flooring.

WOOD POLISHES AND WAXES

Wood needs special attention to maintain its beauty, a fact which has been appreciated for centuries. The much-admired, heavily carved chairs and tables in medieval halls would not look so good today without wax. However, in the past only beeswax, with hardly any additives, would have been used. Industrially-produced furniture polishes are totally different. Especially with modern furniture sprays, there are some questionable additives and preservatives to be found, which increase the shine of wooden surfaces, but are not exactly beneficial for the health of the inhabitants of this shiny home. Luckily, easy-to-make and healthy wood care is available to all, and wood polishes and waxes can be made without much effort.

FRAGRANT BEESWAX POLISH

100g pure beeswax blocks
100ml fine edible oil (olive or rapeseed oil)
10 drops essential citrus oil

The beeswax blocks are melted in a bain marie (water bath). As soon as the wax is completely melted, remove it from its water bath and slowly stir in the oil, then the essential citrus oil. Stir well and pour into a sealable tin container or screw-top jar. From there spread on a soft cloth and polish the wooden surfaces with it in circular movements. Then polish with a dry cloth.

CLASSIC BEESWAX POLISH

250g pure beeswax blocks
100ml turpentine
100ml water
50ml lemon juice
50g grated curd soap

Place the beeswax blocks in a suitable pyrex or glass bowl of sufficient size, place it in a large pan of water, heat it gently and melt the beeswax in this water bath. As soon as the wax has melted evenly, remove it from the water bath and slowly and carefully stir in the turpentine (please use genuine turpentine, not a substitute for turpentine).

Put to one side. The freshly squeezed lemon juice is poured through a coffee filter and mixed with the 100g water. Let this mixture boil briefly in a saucepan, then stir in the soap flakes. Continue stirring until the soap is completely dissolved. Pour the lemon juice mixture very slowly into the beeswax mixture, stirring constantly until an even mixture is obtained. Then pour it all into a tin container with a tight lid or a screw-top glass jar and let it cool completely before closing.

This classic wax polish is correctly applied by dipping a soft cloth into the polish and distributing a small amount of it in circular movements on the wooden surface. The wood is then dry-polished with a second cloth.

CLASSIC BEESWAX POLISH

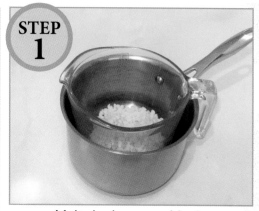

Melt the beeswax blocks
in a water bath.

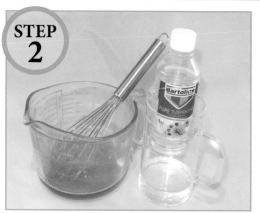

Stir in the turpentine and
set to one side.

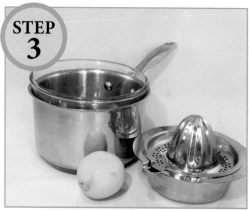

Add the lemon juice through a coffee
filter. Bring to the boil with the water.

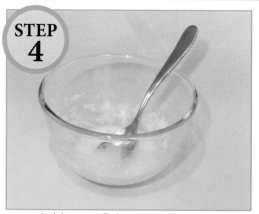

Add soap flakes and stir until
completely dissolved.

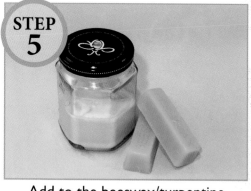

Add to the beeswax/turpentine
mixture and stir well. Fill into a screw-
top jar and close only after cooling.

QUICK POLISH WITH ROSEMARY SCENT

100ml linseed oil
10 drops essential rosemary oil

This polish is intended for immediate use. Mix the essential rosemary oil with the linseed oil in a suitable bowl. The polish is gently applied to the wooden surface with a soft brush and then rubbed into the wood with a soft cloth in circular movements. Then wipe in circular movements with a dry cloth until the wood surface is completely dry.

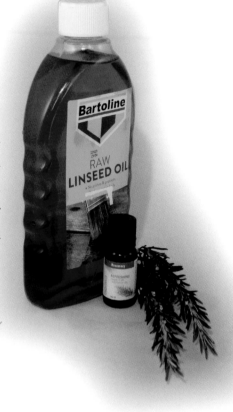

NOURISHING POLISH WITH CARNAUBA WAX

50g carnauba wax flakes
100ml linseed oil
10 drops essential lavender oil

Sometimes also known as Brazil wax, it can be produced sustainably. The carnauba wax flakes and linseed oil are placed in a heatproof jug or bowl. Place in a water bath and heat slowly, stirring frequently until the wax has completely dissolved in the oil. Remove from the water bath, stir in the essential lavender oil then stir the whole

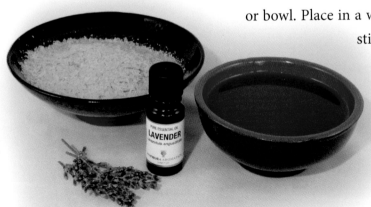

thing again thoroughly. Finally, the cooling wax is poured into a sealable tin can or screw-top jar. Do not close until it has cooled down completely!

Carnauba wax is the hardest natural wax. Mixed with linseed oil, it becomes one of the best wood care preservatives available. This nourishing paste is applied with a dry cloth in small circular movements. Then polish carefully with a second, dry cloth.

BEESWAX WITH LEMON

150ml linseed oil
50ml lemon juice
50g beeswax in flakes
50g carnauba wax in flakes
20 drops essential citrus oil

Put the linseed oil, the beeswax flakes, the carnauba wax flakes and the freshly squeezed and filtered lemon juice into a heatproof bowl and heat slowly in a water bath, stirring frequently. When the wax is completely melted, stir in the essential oil. Then remove the bowl and pour the mixture into a round tin container with a smooth rim. As soon as the melt has cooled down a little, place the container in the fridge. Once the wax has set, it can be used to coat the wooden floor, then rubbed in firmly with a cloth. Polish with a dry cloth.

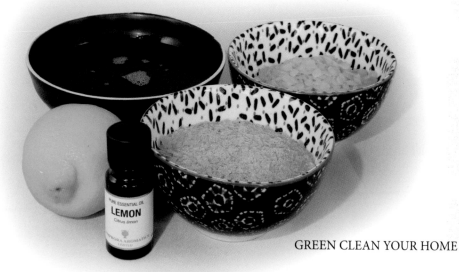

WALNUT POLISH FOR DARK WOOD

100ml walnut oil
100ml linseed oil
100ml lemon juice

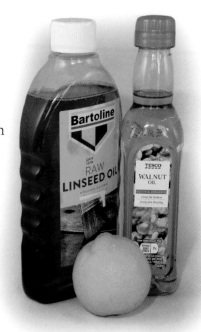

The freshly squeezed lemon juice is poured through a coffee filter, mixed well with the two oils and poured into a sealable container. Apply a thin layer of the polish with a soft brush to the wooden surface, rub it into the wood with a soft cloth in circular movements then wipe thoroughly with a dry cloth. This polish is especially suitable for darker woods.

If you want to produce a larger quantity of this polish for future use, use essential citrus oil instead of fresh lemon juice, which has a limited shelf life of about a month, whereas the essential citrus oil version lasts for months and months.

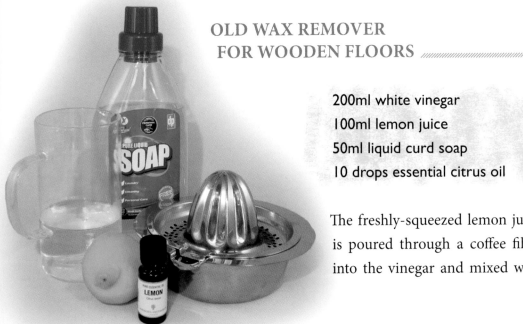

OLD WAX REMOVER FOR WOODEN FLOORS

200ml white vinegar
100ml lemon juice
50ml liquid curd soap
10 drops essential citrus oil

The freshly-squeezed lemon juice is poured through a coffee filter into the vinegar and mixed with the liquid soap and essential citrus oil. Then you pour the whole thing into a bucket big enough to dip your mop into. Now the wooden floor is wiped with strong, short strokes. It makes sense to divide the floor area into small sections and dry each section immediately after with a floor cloth.

This wax remover is suitable for unsealed wooden floors from which you need to remove the dirty old wax layer before polishing it with fresh wax.

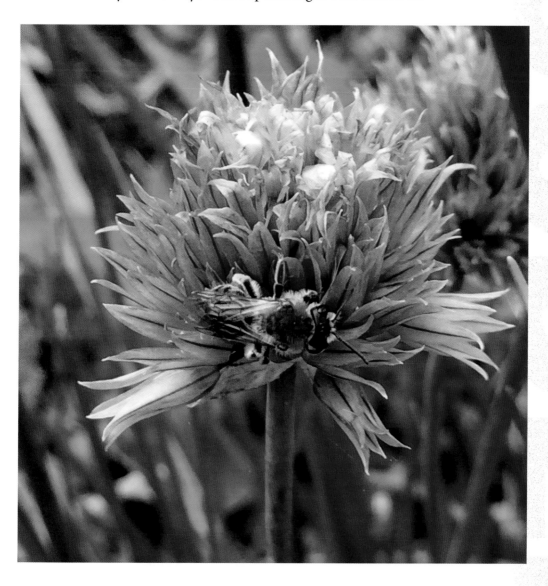

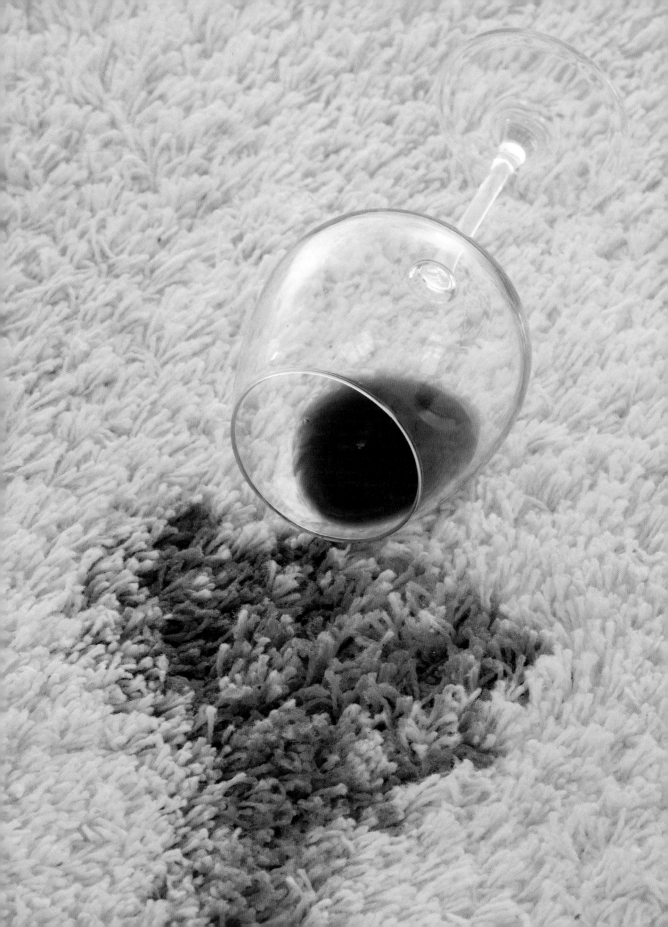

CHAPTER EIGHT

CARPETS

A CARPET GIVES WARMTH TO A LIVING SPACE AND IS AN IMPORTANT DECORATIVE ELEMENT. BUT IT ALSO ALLOWS PLENTY OF SCOPE FOR THE ACCUMULATION OF DIRT

Carpets create a living space of comfort and warmth. But they also absorb a lot of dirt. In addition, there are house dust mites and, if you have dogs or cats, sometimes fleas and their eggs. This is not only unhealthy, but the micro-organisms also ruin the carpet.

Cleaning with a vacuum cleaner removes the coarse dirt. However, frequently-used areas should be pre-cleaned with a broom before vacuuming, and the pile loosened. This allows the deeper-lying dirt to come to the surface to be removed with the vacuum cleaner. An upright vacuum cleaner is ideal for carpet cleaning.

Modern carpets are often coated on the underside, to prevent slipping on smooth floors, and to prevent dirt from falling through the carpet.

But sometimes the carpet needs a proper deep cleaning, a carpet shampoo, which removes deep stains, loosens the fibres and refreshes the colours. This can be done by one of the numerous carpet shampoo specialist firms but you risk the carpet being soaked with a chemical cocktail. Better still, do it yourself, just as well, with homemade products.

Soap is a good base for carpet cleaning products. It has a slightly moisturising effect, so that the textile fibres of the carpet do not dry out too much. New soiling cannot then adhere so easily to the fibres. It is also possible to protect wool carpets against moths by adding essential cedar or lavender oil to the cleaning solution. However, when wet cleaning a carpet, be careful not to do too much of a good thing. A very light foam with little soap, applied in the form of a carpet shampoo, is far more effective than soaking the carpet in a rich soap broth.

Some general rules for the care of carpets to keep the cleaning effort to a minimum

CARPET FRINGES can be tidied straight with the vacuum cleaner's crevice nozzle. Hover the nozzle about two centimetres away from the fringe. It is also possible to spray the fringes with starch (but first put some paper under them!) to give them more hold.

RUGS, RUNNERS AND SMALL CARPETS can be cleaned with a carpet beater, as of old. But not too often, because this type of cleaning puts a lot of strain on the fabric. Carpets made of natural fibres such as sisal, rushes or coconut should not be beaten at all, but only vacuumed. If they need a thorough cleaning, it is best to wash them in salt water and then dry them in the open air.

'WALKING ROUTES' are heavily-used areas on a rug. Not only do they become particularly dirty, they also soon show signs of wear. This can largely be avoided by turning the rug so that it is evenly worn in all directions.

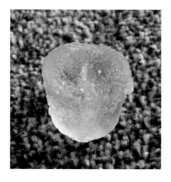

PRESSURE MARKS on a carpet disappear when you melt an ice cube on the indent. Then dab off the water and allow the area to dry thoroughly.

CIGARETTE SMOKE clings to curtains, upholstered furniture and carpets. A bowl of water in the room, preferably with a dash of vinegar, reduces the lingering smell. A lit candle can also remove the smell of tobacco smoke.

FOOD AND DRINK STAINS should be treated as quickly as possible. First dab them with towels or kitchen roll to absorb as much of the liquid as possible. Do not rub, as this will only force the stain deeper into the pile. Remaining traces of the stain can be gently removed with a solution of vinegar and a little soap or bicarbonate of soda.

BLOOD STAINS should be dabbed with cold water immediately. If the stain cannot be completely removed, it can be dabbed with a cloth moistened with cold water and a few drops of essential eucalyptus oil.

MUD STAINS should be sprinkled with salt or bicarbonate of soda or a mixture of both. Let the salt or powder soak in for about an hour. When the damp stain is dried it can easily be vacuumed off, together with the salt or powder.

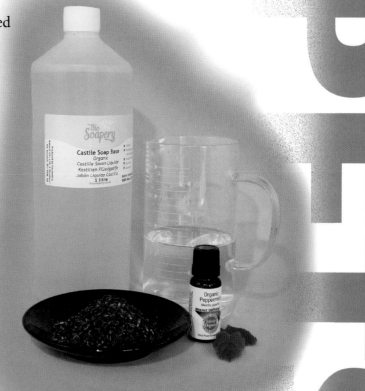

INK STAINS are first sprinkled with cream of tartar and left to take effect. Then take half a lemon, squeeze a few drops of lemon juice onto the stain and then rub the flesh over it. Finally brush away the cream of tartar and remove the lemon juice and any remaining fruit flesh with a damp sponge.

URINE STAINS, usually those from puppies and kittens, are first dabbed with paper towels to absorb as much of the liquid as possible. Then mix 100ml vinegar with 10ml liquid soap and ten drops of essential citrus oil, apply this mixture with a sponge to the affected area of the carpet and let it work for about half an hour. Vinegar and essential citrus oil not only dissolve the urine stain, they also disinfect it and eliminate the odour. Finally, dab the area dry with a soft cloth.

STAIN REMOVER FOR CARPETS

STAIN REMOVER POWDER FOR CARPETS

20g washing soda
20g citric acid powder
Some hot water

Washing soda and citric acid powder are mixed well together. Sprinkle this mixture on the stain and rub a little so that the powder penetrates as deeply as possible into the pile. Allow to work in a little, then pour a little hot water over it, rub carefully and gently as the solution foams, then dab with a sponge.

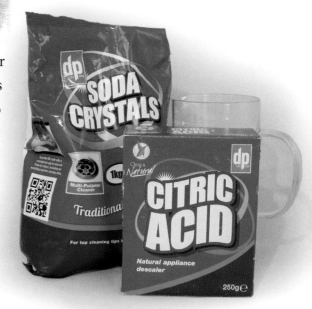

CARPET SHAMPOO WITH PEPPERMINT

10g dried peppermint leaves
250ml boiling water
100ml liquid curd soap
        or Castile liquid soap
10 drops essential peppermint oil

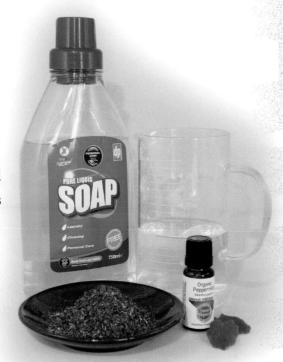

Pour the boiling water over the dried and finely chopped peppermint leaves in a suitable bowl or pan. Allow to stand for about a quarter of an hour, then strain into a bowl and mix with the liquid soap until a smooth solution is obtained. Then stir in the essential peppermint oil.

Rub this shampoo into the carpet with a sponge and allow the foam to dry completely. It can then be vacuumed with a vacuum cleaner.

FOAM CLEANER FOR CARPETS

100ml liquid soap
200ml water
30g bicarbonate of soda
20 drops essential citrus oil

The liquid soap is stirred into the water until an even soap solution is obtained. Then stir in the soda powder and the essential oil. This shampoo is used to foam up on the carpet and is rinsed off with clear water. Then let the carpet dry well.

POWERFUL CARPET WASHING SOLUTION

2 litres hot water
50g alum powder
100ml white vinegar essence
10 drops essential citrus or rosemary oil

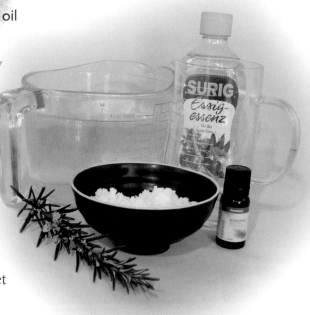

The alum powder is completely dissolved in hot water in a suitable bucket. Then stir in the vinegar essence and the essential oil. You then dip a sponge mop into the carpet shampoo, squeeze out the excess liquid and gently wipe the carpet clean. Rinse the sponge mop clean in a second bucket of clear water before dipping it into the bucket of washing solution again.

The mixture of vinegar and alum cleanses and loosens the carpet fibres, and the essential oil leaves a discreet, fresh scent.

CARPET POWDER FRESHENER

150g bicarbonate of soda
100g fine cornflour
15 drops essential juniper oil
10 drops essential cedar oil

Bicarbonate of soda and cornflour are mixed well together in a suitable bowl then sprinkled with the essential oils. Because the cornflour easily forms lumps with the drops of essential oils, the mixture must be stirred very carefully. Once all the lumps have been dispersed by stirring, the powder can be sprinkled over the carpet. It should be left to work for several hours before being vacuumed up.

This product is particularly suitable if the carpet already emits a certain musty smell from pets or children's bare feet. This deodorant makes the smell disappear. The carpet smells fresh again and it looks it!

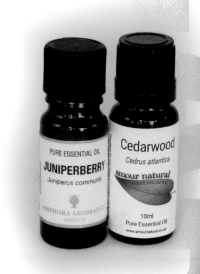

ROSEMARY CARPET SHAMPOO

10g dried rosemary
250ml boiling water
50g bicarbonate of soda
30g soap flakes or grated curd soap
15 drops essential rosemary oil

Pour the boiling water over the dried rosemary in a suitable pan. Allow to steep for about a quarter of an hour, then strain into a bowl and mix first with the soap flakes, then with the bicarbonate of soda and finally the essential rosemary oil. The shampoo is applied with a sponge to the carpet and rubbed carefully until it foams. Using a bucket of clean water, the sponge is wrung out and the carpet sponged again several times. Finally let the foam dry and then vacuum it away.

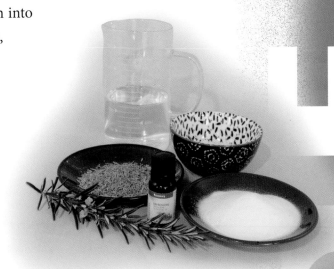

ANTI-FLEA POWDER FOR CARPETS

250g bicarbonate of soda
10 drops essential citrus oil
10 drops essential peppermint oil
10 drops essential tea tree oil

The bicarbonate of soda is sprinkled with the essential oils and mixed thoroughly so that the oils are evenly distributed in the powder. First the carpet is thoroughly vacuumed, then the powder is sprinkled on the carpet and left to work for at least an hour. Then vacuum the powder thoroughly with a vacuum cleaner and immediately throw the vacuum cleaner bag into the rubbish. There will be many dead and dying fleas and their eggs in it.

Of course, one should also give the pet an anti-flea treatment.

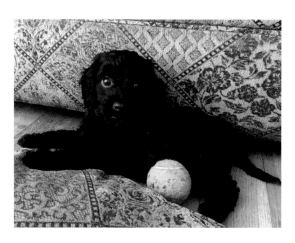

ANTIBACTERIAL CARPET SPRAY

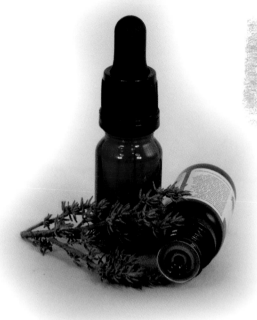

20g dried thyme
300ml boiling water
100ml white vinegar
50g bicarbonate of soda
20 drops essential thyme oil

Pour the boiling water over the dried thyme in a suitable bowl or pan. Cover and leave to stand for about quarter of an hour, then strain into a bowl, mix with vinegar, the soda powder and finally the essential thyme oil. As always, when bicarbonate of soda meets the vinegar, it foams. The container should therefore be large enough to avoid foaming over. After cooling, decant into a spray bottle.

This antibacterial liquid can be sprayed onto the carpet and left to dry. The mixture is also suitable for use in shampoo vacuum cleaners. Depending on the size of the tank of the device, the appropriate amount of this cleaner can be produced; just stick to the proportions of the ingredients.

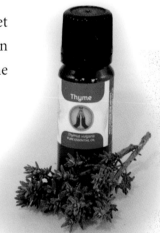

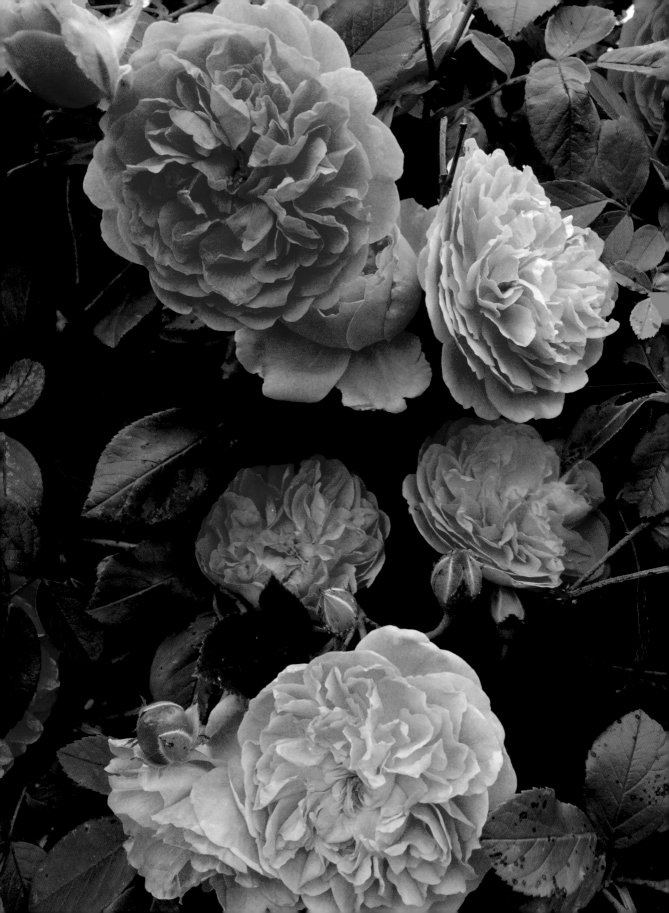

CHAPTER NINE

AIR FRESHENERS AND ROOM SPRAYS

SUPERMARKETS OFFER A WIDE RANGE OF PRODUCTS TO IMPROVE THE SMELL OF A ROOM. BUT WHAT *ARE* THE INGREDIENTS? YOU MIGHT PREFER TO MAKE THESE AIR FRESHENERS YOURSELF

AIR FRESHENERS

For hundreds of years, air fresheners have played an important role in the home. With their help, it was possible to mask the often unpleasant odours caused by poor hygiene conditions. Today we have pretty good hygiene, but we now have other sources of unwanted smells. Anyone who has ever assembled a cupboard knows how long it can give off a penetrating smell of solvents into the room. Carpets, curtains or freshly painted walls can also produce toxic vapours from volatile organic compounds such as formaldehyde or trichloroethylene. If the smell becomes weaker over time, it can mean the problem is simply below the perception level of our sense of smell.

Indoor plants offer us a means of air purification. They create a kind of air filter because they constantly absorb carbon dioxide and pollutants from the air and convert them into oxygen through photosynthesis. This filter function of indoor plants may well be sufficient for an averagely-polluted living environment with older furnishings. However, it should be remembered that plants need a lot of light to perform this function. If you can offer them this, you can choose from a whole range of special 'filter plants': Spider plant (*Chlorophytum comosum vittatum*), Devil's ivy (*Epipremnum aureum*), Weeping fig (*Ficus benjamina*), Chinese evergreen (*Aglaonema modestum*), to name but a few. Those who fill their windowsills with herb pots and windowboxes will have, besides all the other pleasures that herbs offer, better indoor air due to the filter function of the herbs. And many herbs also have a very pleasant fragrance, which makes them a living air freshener.

POTPOURRIS

Dozens of fragrant herbs open up endless possibilities of different fragrance combinations. You can create your own individual room scent, experiment again and again and simply feel good in your discreetly-scented living environment. In contrast to the countless industrially-produced room sprays and evaporators of synthetic aromatic oils, potpourris are not an additional source of toxic air pollutants. They do not evaporate benzene, toluene or formaldehyde. They create well-being and not, like industrial products, headaches, asthma or allergies. The essential oils of dried herbs – which in some cases can also have an allergenic effect – are released into the air in such small quantities that they hardly ever irritate the immune system of very sensitive people. Also, the choice of dried herbs is not limited to those that grow in your own garden, balcony or windowsill.

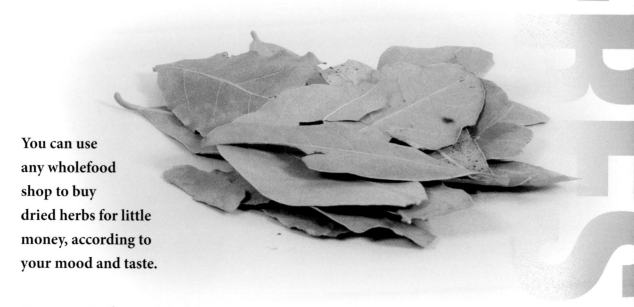

You can use any wholefood shop to buy dried herbs for little money, according to your mood and taste.

Potpourris from dried herbs need a fixative to preserve the essential oils of the various herbs and flowers for a longer period of time. As a fixative you can use woody plant parts, such as pine cones or cedar wood shavings, but most easily you can use the dried, powdered rhizomes of the iris – orris powder – also because this powder is very easy to use. Oak moss, calamus root, benzoin resin, incense, cinnamon sticks and patchouli leaves are also used.

The potpourri itself can be put together from various dried herbs, flowers, leaves, stems, from powdered or finely chopped root parts, from dried fruit peels and also from spices such as ginger, nutmeg or cloves. The possibilities are limited only by your personal taste.

As additional fragrances, use matching essential oils. They prolong the time in which the potpourri exudes its scent. Of course, the essential oils can also be used to make very exotic fragrance mixtures. However, those who value a harmonious, unobtrusive room fragrance should choose essential oils that correspond to the herbs and flowers used.

Making a potpourri is very easy. And if you can't get the dried herbs and flowers from your own garden or balcony, you can buy them easukt. Dried flowers are also available in many handicraft shops.

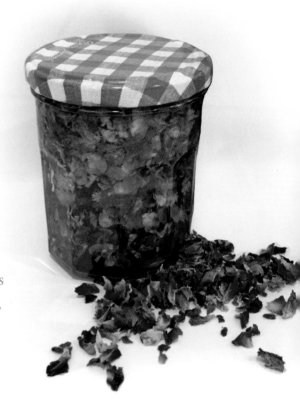

The dried herbs and flowers are placed in a screw-top jar of a suitable size, sparingly sprinkled with the selected essential oil and sprinkled with the fixative such as orris root powder. Then you close the jar, shake it vigorously and place it out of direct sunlight. The jar is shaken at least once a day. It takes a minimum of four weeks, depending on the ingredients, for the fragrance to develop fully.

During this 'maturing period' shake the glass daily. Then tip the contents into a suitable small bowl, place it away from the heater and out of direct sunlight, and enjoy the scent of the potpourri for weeks.

There are countless recipes for potpourris, so here are some to serve as an inspiration for your own creations. You can follow them for your first attempts, or as a base from which to expand, according to your personal taste.

POTPOURRI ////////////////////////////////////

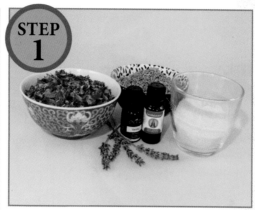

STEP 1

All the ingredients you need.

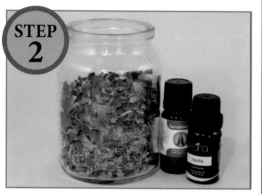

STEP 2

The dried flowers are poured loosely into a sealable jar and drizzled with essential oil.

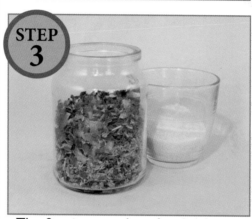

STEP 3

The fixative powder of violet (orris) root is shaken over it.

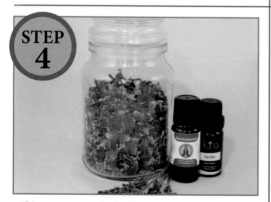

STEP 4

Close jar and shake thoroughly. Then you put it in a cool place for about four weeks. Shake every day.

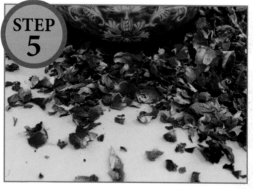

STEP 5

After the 'maturing period' the potpourri is ready to perfume the living space for weeks with its fragrance.

DISCREET ROMANTIC FRAGRANCE

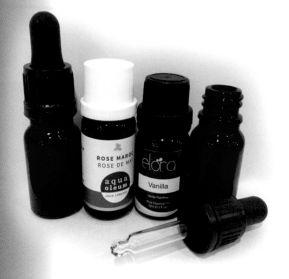

10g dried rose petals

10g lavender flowers, dried

10g dried geranium leaves

10g orris (violet) root, finely ground

5g lemon verbena leaves, dried

10 drops essential vanilla oil

5 drops essential sandalwood oil

This potpourri spreads a sweet, romantic fragrance without being too obvious. When putting it together, be careful not to use too much of the essential sandalwood oil. It blends harmoniously into the fragrance composition in the specified quantity. If you use too much of it, it can mask other scents.

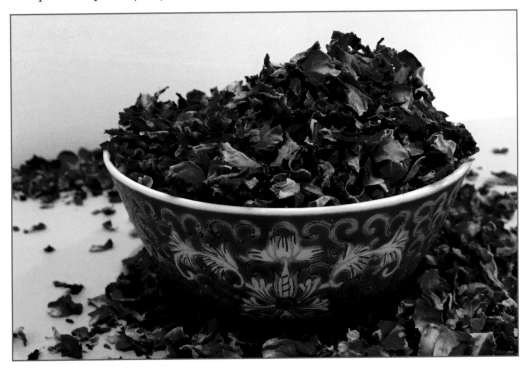

SPRING FRAGRANCE FOR WINTER DAYS

10g rosemary leaves, dried
10g mint leaves, dried
5g dried thyme leaves
5g cloves whole
lemon peel, grated
orange peel, grated
10 drops essential orange oil

In this recipe, the grated lemon and orange peel acts as a fixative. This potpourri spreads a subtle scent of spring to help you to cope with those melancholy feelings, especially on late winter days, and fills you with hope of the approaching spring.

SOOTHING FRAGRANCE MIXTURE

10g dried clover flowers
10g camomile flowers, dried
10g lavender flowers, dried
5g dill stems, dried
5g lemon balm leaves, dried
5g orris (violet) root, dried and finely ground
10 drops essential camomile oil

This potpourri exudes a calming fragrance. It is therefore not only suitable as a fragrance for the living room and bedroom of nervous people, but also as the filling for a fragrance pillow on their beds. It contributes to a calm, healthy sleep.

RUSTIC SCENT OF APPLES AND HERBS

5 dried apple slices, quartered
10g lavender flowers, dried
10g bay leaves, dried
10g sage leaves, dried
10g ginger root, dried and finely ground
2 cinnamon sticks, broken into small pieces
10 drops essential lavender oil

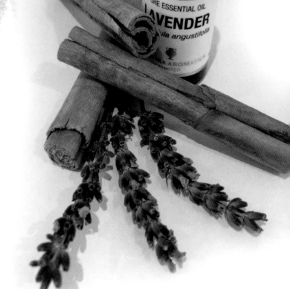

This fragrance is reminiscent of a late summer day in the country. The dried apple slices not only contribute their scent to the mixture, but also act as a fixative. This potpourri works well in a bowl as a dispenser of room scent, and also in a linen bag between the clothes in the wardrobe.

SPICY-FRESH ORANGE SCENT

15g marigold blossoms, dried
10g calamus root (orris powder), dried and finely ground
grated peel of two oranges
3 dried and quartered apple slices
15 drops essential orange oil

This mixture results in a spicy potpourri which is also well suited for scented bags. Calamus root and apple slices not only contribute their scents to the potpourri, but also act as fixatives.

FRESH SUMMER SCENT

10g basil, dried
10g camomile, dried
10g marjoram, dried
5g yarrow, dried
5 halved juniper berries
some dried oakmoss
grated orange peel
5g orris root as fixative
15 drops essential cedar oil

The scent of this potpourri is reminiscent of summer gardens and meadows. You can put it in a bowl and fill the living room with it. But it also goes well in a scented pillow, or you can sew it into a linen bag, hang it in the wardrobe and transfer the summer scent to your clothes.

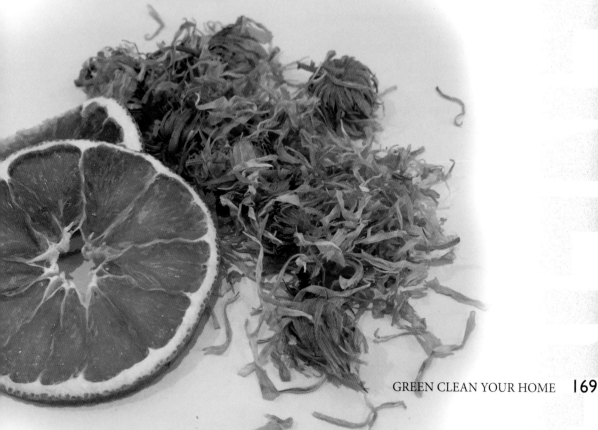

SENSUAL FRAGRANCE MIXTURE //

15g jasmine blossoms, dried
15g lemon verbena leaves, dried
10g ginger root, finely ground in mortar
10g muscat sage leaves, dried
5g cumin seed
3 tonka beans
1 vanilla pod, cut into small pieces
20 drops essential patchouli oil

This fragrance composition with a top note of vanilla leads to sensual dreams. It takes about six weeks to develop its full fragrance in a sealed screw-top jar with plenty of extensive daily shaking.

The tonka beans listed in the ingredients are available in health food shops and via mail order. They are tasteless legumes with a strong vanilla-like aroma. This potpourri also works as a fragrance cushion or a fragrance bag in the wardrobe.

ROOM SPRAYS WITH FRESH HERBAL SCENT

If you don't want to make a potpourri and wait four to six weeks for its fragrance to mature, you can make your own immediately-effective room spray as an alternative. This room spray is designed to quickly eliminate unpleasant odours. All you need is distilled water and a collection of essential oils according to your personal preferences. Distilled water is recommended because the minerals in tap water *may* react with some essential oils and thus reduce their fragrance potential.

For a room spray, mix about ten drops of an essential oil with a quarter of a litre of distilled water and fill the whole thing into a spray bottle. Shake the bottle thoroughly before each use, because the essential oils should always be evenly distributed in the solution.

Spray directly into the air, and you can also spray curtains and carpets with it. These solutions should not be sprayed directly on human skin, where they can cause irritation, even if you are not allergic to any of the essential oils used.

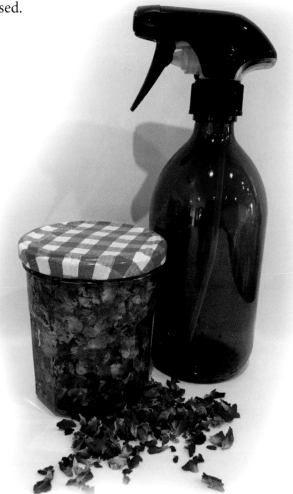

You can eliminate unpleasant smells with the spread of spicy, romantic or soothing fragrances – there are hardly any limits to the imagination. Which essential oils you combine into which fragrance composition is entirely up to you.

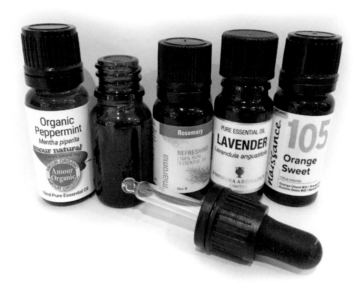

Here are some ideas:

SPICY RUSTIC SCENT

Rose, geranium, rosemary, orange, cinnamon, ginger, vanilla, laurel

SOOTHING EARTHY FRAGRANCE

Bergamot, geranium, patchouli, thyme, sage, cedar, incense, clary sage, camomile, yarrow

ROMANTIC FRAGRANCE

Vanilla, rose, neroli, jasmine, sandalwood

STIMULATING AND CONCENTRATION-PROMOTING FRAGRANCE

Basil, rosemary, lavender, orange, nutmeg, peppermint, lime, coriander

FRESH PETAL ROOM SPRAY

If you have fresh rose petals or lavender blossoms to hand, you can make a particularly fine room spray. To do this, the fresh flowers or petals are placed in a screw top jar and poured over with distilled water. The jar should be full to the brim. Then close it up and put it in the blazing sun all day long. By evening, the water will have mixed with the essential oils of the flowers and will exude their scent in a subtle way.

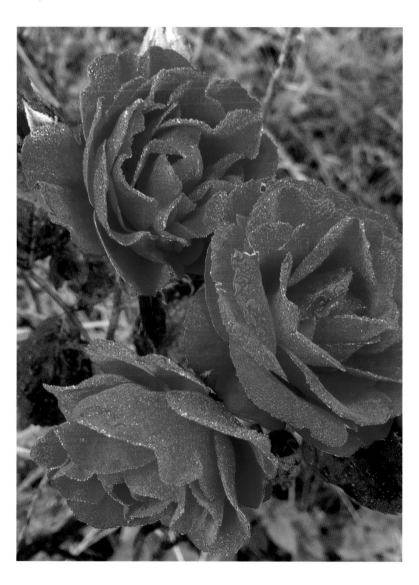

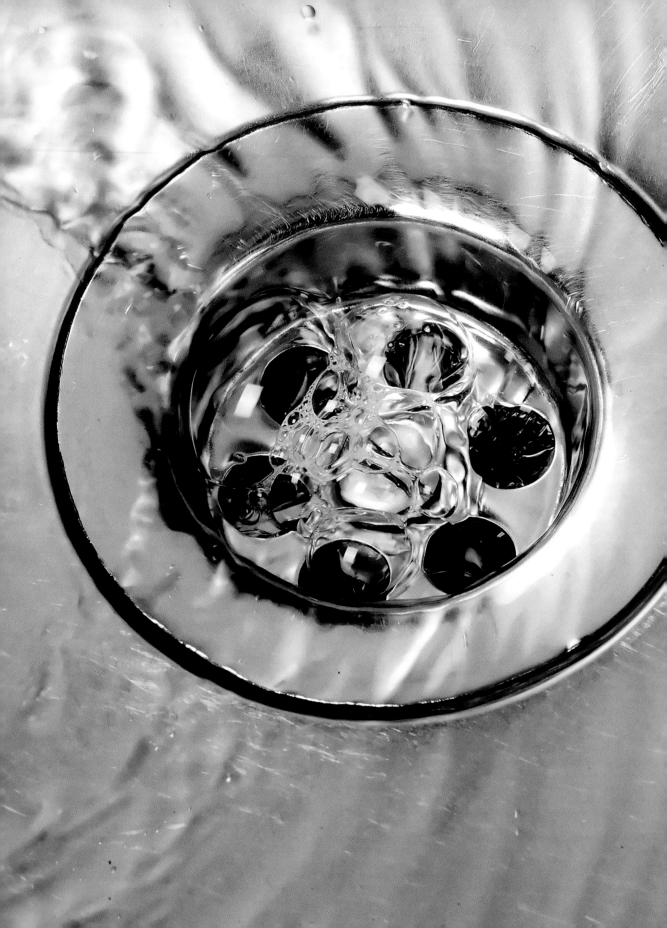

CHAPTER TEN

CLEANING AGENTS FOR METALS

METALS CAN POSE A CHALLENGE WHEN IT COMES TO CLEANING THEM, BUT HERE'S HOW TO DO IT RIGHT

Metals tend to form stains that are often very difficult to remove. No matter whether it's door handles made of brass or anodized metals, parts of furniture, floor lamps or silverware – many today believe that metals can only be cleaned and polished with metal cleaners available on the market. You can prove them wrong with these homemade metal cleaners. In addition, you can avoid combining various strong acids, which in the long run are bad for the metal and also bad for the environment.

Homemade metal cleaners may not immediately achieve the penetrating effect of those available commercially. But with just a little more elbow grease, they are just as good. And you can be sure you aren't contaminating your indoor air with unwanted molecules. What you actually need for a harmless form of metal cleaning is usually already in your kitchen.

CHROME

... is a bright, shiny and very hard metal with which many other metals are coated. The surfaces of kitchen appliances or taps are often chrome plated. These should not be cleaned with scouring agents, as this can scratch the thin chromium layer and make it porous.

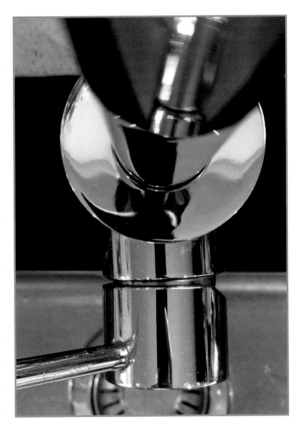

If no stubborn stains are to be removed, it is usually sufficient to rub them with vinegar on a soft cloth and then polish them with a dry cloth.

In the event of stubborn stains such as those from burnt-on fat, several drops of essential eucalyptus oil are applied to a cloth and the stains will rub off. Then wipe the area dry with a clean cloth.

ALUMINIUM

... is the most common metal in the earth's crust. Because it mostly occurs as a silicate compound and because its extraction is very complex, it is usually smelted out of bauxite. Bare aluminium surfaces very quickly form an oxide layer when in contact with air. This protects the metal from corrosion. Aluminium does not tarnish, but reacts very easily with certain substances. Therefore, it should not be cleaned with homemade detergents containing bicarbonate of soda or washing soda. Stains on aluminium surfaces can however be removed very easily with one of the following cleaning agents.

LEMON PASTE FOR ALUMINIUM

Mix half a cup of white vinegar, three tablespoons of cream of tartar and a few drops of essential citrus oil to make a smooth paste. This is applied to the aluminium surface to be cleaned and left to act briefly. Then rub the surface clean with a cloth and wipe thoroughly with a wet cloth.

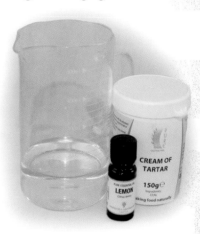

CORNFLOUR AND ALUM PASTE FOR ALUMINIUM

Mix two tablespoons of cornflour, two tablespoons of alum powder and five drops of essential citrus oil with a teaspoon at a time of warm water, to form a smooth paste. This is used to rub the aluminium surface until it is clean. Then rinse the paste off with water and dry the surface.

VINEGAR CITRUS WASHING-UP LIQUID FOR ALUMINIUM DISHES ////////////////////////

This special washing-up liquid is ideal for aluminium dishes. Mix a quarter of a litre of water with an eighth of a litre of white vinegar and ten drops of essential citrus oil. Soak the aluminium dishes in a little water, add this mixture and top up with more water until the dishes are completely covered. Leave to soak for about an hour, then rinse clean and dry.

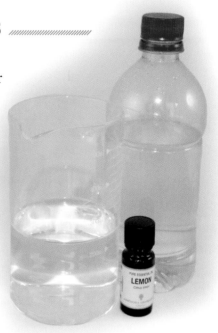

BRASS

... is an alloy of copper and zinc. As with copper, brass ornaments are usually coated with a colourless lacquer to protect them from corrosion. In this case, it is sufficient to dust the items and wipe them with a damp cloth from time to time. Older brass objects do not have this protective layer and as a result they assume a greenish tinge in time. It's rather beautiful – think of the Statue of Liberty – but if you don't want to look at this patina and you prefer shiny brass, then here are some harmless means to achieve this.

SALT PASTE

Mix two tablespoons of salt and a few drops of essential citrus oil in a cup of vinegar and add enough flour to make a thick paste. This is then applied to the brass surface and rubbed with a dry sponge. Allow the paste to dry and rinse with warm water. Then rub the surface dry and polish it with a soft cloth.

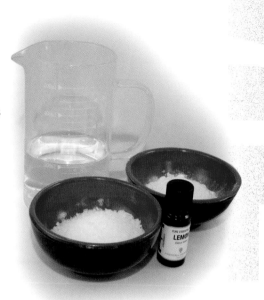

MILK BATH

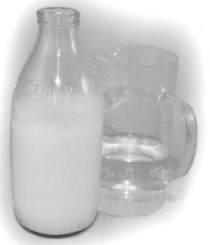

... contains lactic acid, and this is a proven solvent for stains on brass. Mix the milk in equal parts with water and place the brass objects in this 'bath' for several hours. Then rinse well, wipe dry and polish with a soft cloth.

TARTAR PASTE

Mix three tablespoons of cream of tartar in half a cup of lemon juice and rub the resulting paste in small circular movements onto the stained brass object. When completely dry, rinse the paste off with water and polish the item dry.

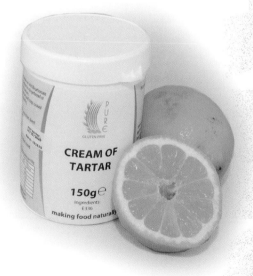

SILVER

In many novels, domestic workers are often busy polishing silverware. If you have silverware but no servants, you probably have to do it yourself. Don't wear rubber gloves for the task! Because silver reacts with rubber, it tarnishes very quickly and can even corrode. Nor is it a good idea to tie silver cutlery together with rubber bands or store it in a rubber-lined box. Very sour dishes tarnish silver. Vinegar, salt, olives, eggs or fruit salads should be eaten with other cutlery.

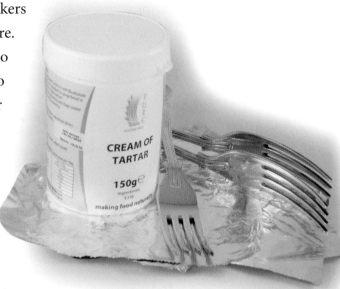

Once the silver has tarnished, it can be made to shine again with a simple but effective remedy. Place the silverware in a bowl filled with water and add three tablespoons of cream of tartar and a few strips of aluminium foil. A chemical reaction then takes place in the bowl, which may also be noticeable by its odour. Hydrogen sulphide is released and this smells like rotten eggs. It is not harmful at these levels, but you should still open the kitchen window. After at least one hour, remove the silver from the water. The silver cutlery, now shiny again, should be thoroughly rinsed with water and then carefully dried.

If silver cutlery cannot be washed up immediately after use, any left over bits of food should be removed completely. And silver cutlery, when not in use, should be rolled up in a clean cloth.

CAST IRON

... is a popular material for frying pans because of its thermal properties. However, it has the disadvantage that it will rust if you do not keep it absolutely dry. Regular care of cast iron pans includes rubbing them with oil. This forms a protective layer against oxidation. A new cast iron pan should first be rubbed gently with a cloth made of fine steel wool and a little soapy water, then dried immediately and coated with a thin layer of vegetable oil on the inside. Place the pan in the oven preheated to 120 °C for about two hours. Then let it cool down, wipe it out with a damp cloth and dry it carefully. This treatment gives the cast iron pan a good protective layer.

A cast iron pan should be cleaned immediately after each use. After washing, oil it, and before the next use wipe off the fat layer with a kitchen cloth. If food remains have burned into the cast iron, they must of course be washed away with a cloth and then washed off with a soapy detergent. After scrubbing, however, the pan has lost its protective layer, so the procedure described above must be repeated with oiling and two hours in the oven.

COPPER

... is a very decorative material. Because it is also susceptible to oxidation, copper ornaments and utensils are usually coated with a thin layer of colourless varnish. This should not be polished, because it could rub off the varnish layer. All you have to do is wipe it with water once in a while.

The situation is different with copper cookware. Stainless steel pans

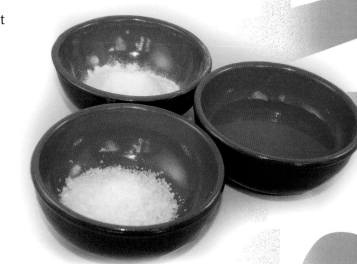

often have a copper base because copper distributes the heat evenly. But whether the whole pan is made of copper or it just has a copper base – the use of scouring agents or steel wool will cause ugly scratches on the copper surface! Only a soft kitchen sponge or a soft cloth should be used for cleaning copper. If the copper tarnishes over time, it can be polished clean with a polishing paste consisting of one part each of salt, flour and vinegar.

For the regular polishing of copper bowls and pans, there are some tried and tested household remedies. You can sprinkle one half of a lemon with salt and rub the copper surfaces with it.

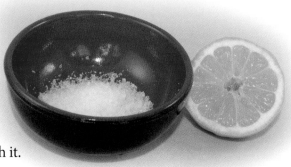

Then wash off with water, polish dry and the copper shines like new.

Or try this polishing paste for copper:

Mix a cup of tomato ketchup with three tablespoons of cream of tartar powder. Spread this paste on the copper surfaces and let it work for about an hour. Then wash the copper part in soapy water and dry it carefully.

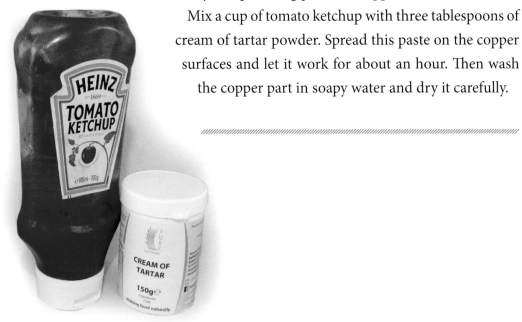

RUST

... is the oxidation product of iron. The best protection against this is to paint iron surfaces or, if this isn't appropriate, to coat it with a little oil. If rust still occurs, it can be dissolved with phosphoric acid or oxalic acid. Rust removers that contain these acids do not have to be bought at a high price. Fresh rhubarb or, if that's not in season, ordinary Cola will do the same.

100g of fresh rhubarb contains 460 mg oxalic acid. The rhubarb stalk is rubbed over the rusty spot and you can literally watch the rust loosen. For heavily-rusted areas, the fresh rhubarb can be pureed and applied directly to the iron or to the grate.

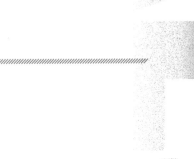

Cola contains up to 15 per cent phosphates, mostly in the form of orthophosphoric acid. If the rusted object is not too big, you can put it in a bowl and pour Cola over it. Leave it to soak for a few hours. Afterwards you can usually simply brush off the rust.

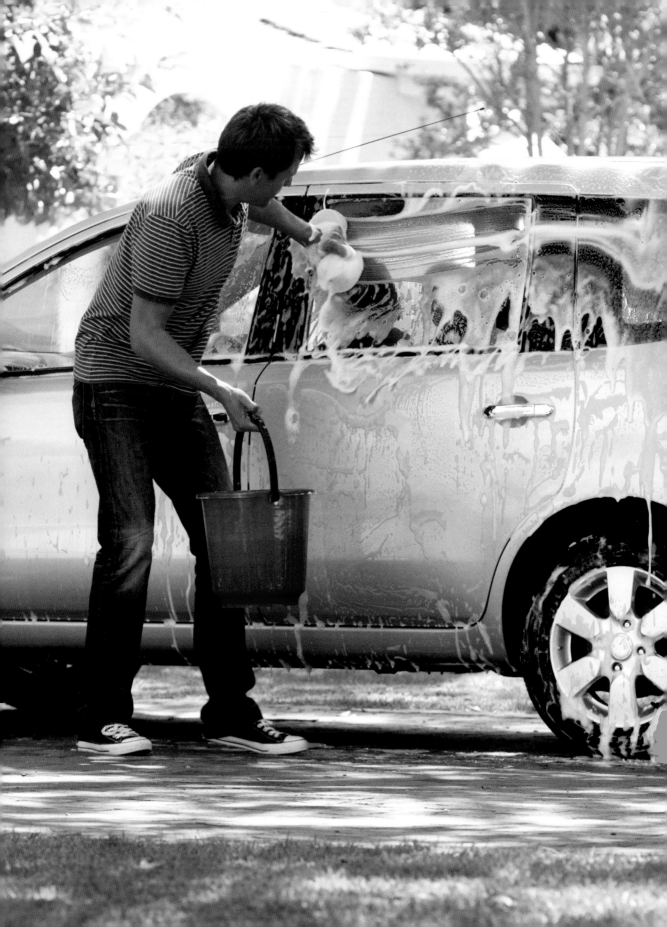

CHAPTER ELEVEN

CAR CLEANING

THINK OF THE CAR AS A ROOM WHERE YOU SPEND A LOT OF TIME. THEREFORE IT SHOULD BE A SPACE WHICH DOES NOT AFFECT YOUR WELL-BEING WITH CHEMICAL SMELLS

CAR WASHING

If you don't have it done at the petrol station, but on your own drive with the garden hose, then you can achieve a good clean with homemade cleaning agents. And of course all the recipes listed are not only suitable for the car, but for boats or caravans too.

SOAP WASH FOR THE CAR

4 litres water
0.5 litres liquid soap
15 drops essential citrus oil

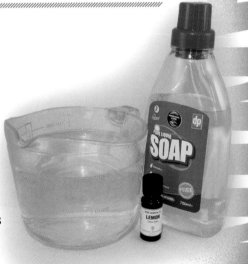

Pour the water into a bucket and stir in first the liquid soap and then the essential oil. The car is washed section by section from top to bottom and each section is rinsed thoroughly with water. This prevents streaks of soap from forming on the paint.

CAR WASH FOR HEAVY SOILING

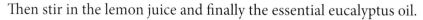

4 litres water
200ml lemon juice
100g bicarbonate of soda
10 drops essential
   eucalyptus oil

The bicarbonate of soda is placed in the bucket with the water. Stir until completely dissolved.
Then stir in the lemon juice and finally the essential eucalyptus oil.

The car is first sprayed with a hose to remove coarse dirt. Then you wash it with a soft sponge using the formula above, in sections from top to bottom – so first the roof, then the bonnet, then the sides. Each section is rinsed thoroughly before moving on to the next.

DETERGENT FOR TYRES

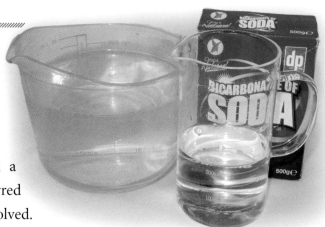

2 litres water
150g bicarbonate of soda
250ml white vinegar

Water and vinegar are mixed in a bucket, then the soda powder is stirred in and mixed until completely dissolved.
This detergent is applied to the tyres with a
sponge or a brush with firm bristles and is brushed off well while still wet. The tyre is then rinsed with water. Such thorough tyre cleaning is particularly appropriate after changing from winter to summer tyres – or vice versa.

WINDSCREEN CLEANERS

GENERAL WINDSCREEN CLEANER

100ml liquid soap
100g bicarbonate of soda
250ml water
10 drops essential eucalyptus oil

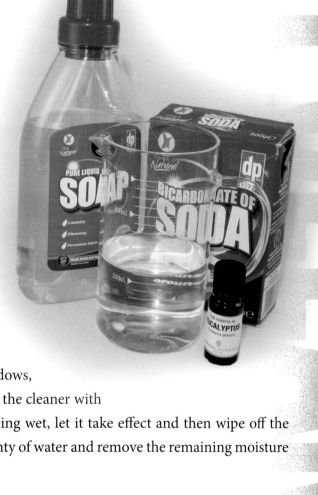

Water and liquid soap are mixed together in a suitable container. Then stir in the bicarbonate of soda until the soap and bicarbonate of soda are completely dissolved in the water. Finally, the essential eucalyptus oil is stirred in.

This windscreen cleaner not only removes dirt and insect remains from the windscreen and other windows, but also from the headlights. Apply the cleaner with a sponge until the window is dripping wet, let it take effect and then wipe off the dirt with the sponge. Wipe with plenty of water and remove the remaining moisture with a rubber wiper.

WINDSCREEN CLEANER FOR THE WINTER

250ml white vinegar
100ml water
20 drops essential citrus oil

All ingredients are mixed well and filled into a spray bottle. This is used to spray onto the windows, wipe them clean with a cloth moistened with the cleaner and remove the remaining moisture with a rubber wiper. This cleaning agent offers not only a clear view but also the advantage that it reduces the formation of frost on the car windows in winter.

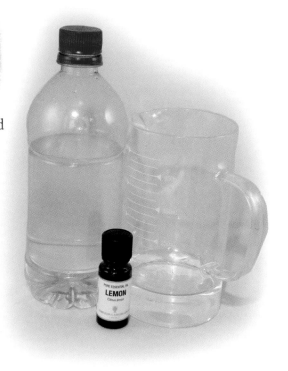

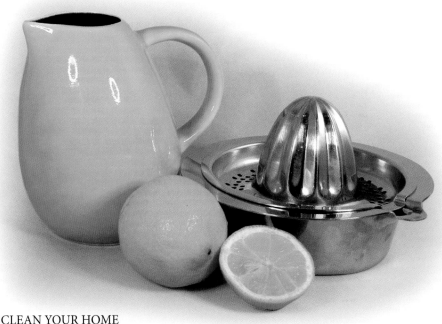

CAR WAX

TWO-PHASE BIO CAR WAX

wax
50g beeswax blocks
50g carnauba wax blocks
100ml linseed oil
10 drops essential citrus oil

Polishing agent
50ml lemon juice

Beeswax, carnauba wax and linseed oil are put into a heat-proof bowl. Place the bowl in a water bath and heat gently, stirring it several times, until a uniform wax melt is obtained. Then add the essential citrus oil, stir again thoroughly and remove the container with the wax melt from the water bath. The mixture is poured immediately into a clean tin container (a metal coffee container is ideal) and, because the container gets hot, don't forget to use oven gloves.

Place the tin can with the melted wax, unsealed, in a cool and dust-free place. In the course of two to three days the wax hardens. It can then easily be removed by tapping on the upturned can. The previously cleaned car is rubbed with this chunk of wax. Allow to work in a little, then dip a clean soft cloth into the freshly squeezed, filtered lemon juice, wring out well and polish the waxed car with it. Finally it is polished to a high gloss with a clean cloth.

UPHOLSTERY CLEANING FOR CARS

VINYL UPHOLSTERY CLEANER

250ml hot water
100g bicarbonate of soda
15 drops essential cedar oil

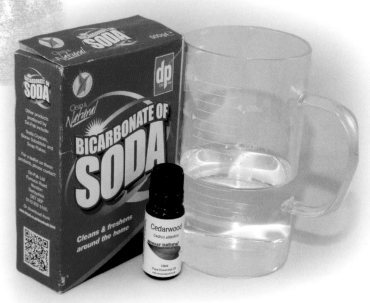

The bicarbonate of soda is completely dissolved in the hot water by stirring. Then mix in the essential cedar oil. First the car seats are cleaned with a vacuum cleaner, not forgetting the cracks and the areas between the seats. Then moisten a soft cloth with the cleaner and rub the seats with it from top to bottom. Finally wipe them dry with a clean cloth.

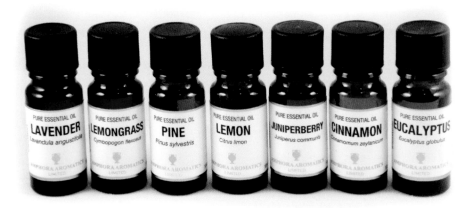

FABRIC UPHOLSTERY CLEANING
WITH SOAPWORT

50g dried and crushed soapwort root
    (from the carnation family)
250ml water

Soapwort root should be soaked in about half a litre of water for several hours before brewing. To brew, pour 250ml of boiling water over the soapwort in a pan and immediately place the pan on the hotplate so that the brew boils for about one minute. Then turn the heat down and let it simmer gently for about 20 minutes, stirring frequently. Now take the pan off the stove and let the decoction continue to brew until it has cooled down. It is then strained and is ready for cleaning textile upholstery.

Dip a brush with very soft bristles into the soapwort liquid and rub it from top to bottom into the fabric seats. Wipe with a dry cloth and let the seats dry in the air.

LEATHER UPHOLSTERY CLEANER

100g soap flakes
150ml hot water
10 drops essential rosemary oil

Completely dissolve the soap flakes
in hot water by stirring thoroughly.
Then stir in the essential rosemary
oil. After hoovering the leather
upholstery, apply this cleaner to the
leather seats with a soft brush in gentle
movements from top to bottom. Then wipe
with a wet cloth and polish the leather parts dry
with a clean cloth. This cleaning agent protects the leather and
at the same time removes all dirt. After cleaning, the leather should be treated with
the following leather spray.

LEATHER CARE SPRAY

100ml olive oil
100ml rosemary extract
50ml white vinegar
5 drops essential rosemary oil

Pour a little more than 100ml of boiling water over
about 10g of dried rosemary. Allow to brew for a good
quarter of an hour and then strain off this strong
decoction. Mix well with olive oil, vinegar and
finally the essential rosemary oil and pour into a
spray bottle when cool. The leather seats are lightly

sprayed with this agent and polished to a high gloss with a soft, dry cloth. The mixture of olive oil and rosemary ensures that the leather always remains soft and does not become porous, even after many years.

DASHBOARD CARE

DASHBOARD QUICK CLEANER

50ml liquid curd soap or Castile liquid soap
150ml hot water
15 drops essential rosemary oil

The liquid soap is completely dissolved in the hot water by stirring. Then stir in the essential rosemary oil and pour the cleaner into a spray bottle. The cleaner is sprayed onto the dashboard, which is then wiped clean with a dry cloth.

This cleaner has the advantage that it is just as suitable for plastics as for textiles and leather. If the dashboard has leather parts, it is recommended to treat them with the leather care spray (*see previous page*).

CARPET AND MAT CARE

CLEANER FOR CARPETS AND MATS

2 litres water
150ml liquid curd soap or Castile liquid soap
15 drops essential rosemary
    or peppermint oil

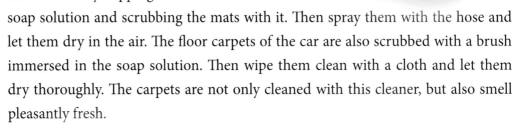

The liquid soap is stirred into the water until completely dissolved. Then stir in the essential oil. First the floor area of the car is carefully cleaned with a vacuum cleaner to remove loose dirt. Then the floor mats are cleaned by dipping a brush into the soap solution and scrubbing the mats with it. Then spray them with the hose and let them dry in the air. The floor carpets of the car are also scrubbed with a brush immersed in the soap solution. Then wipe them clean with a cloth and let them dry thoroughly. The carpets are not only cleaned with this cleaner, but also smell pleasantly fresh.

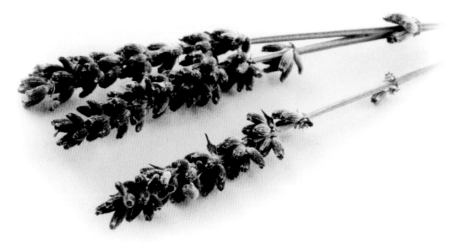

AIR FRESHENER

AIR FRESHENER FOR THE CAR

200ml distilled water
50ml white vinegar
10 drops essential lavender oil
10 drops essential orange oil

Distilled water and vinegar are mixed, then the essential oils are stirred in and the whole thing is filled into a spray bottle. As soon as the interior of the car begins to smell a bit stale – usually after a rainy day or when a four-legged friend spreads out on the back seat – upholstery and floor covering are sprayed sparingly with this spray from a distance of around 20 centimetres. After spraying, the car should be well ventilated. Yes, and the dog should not jump straight back into the car, because the fresh essential oils could irritate his nose and paws!

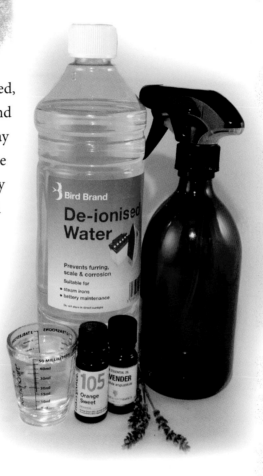

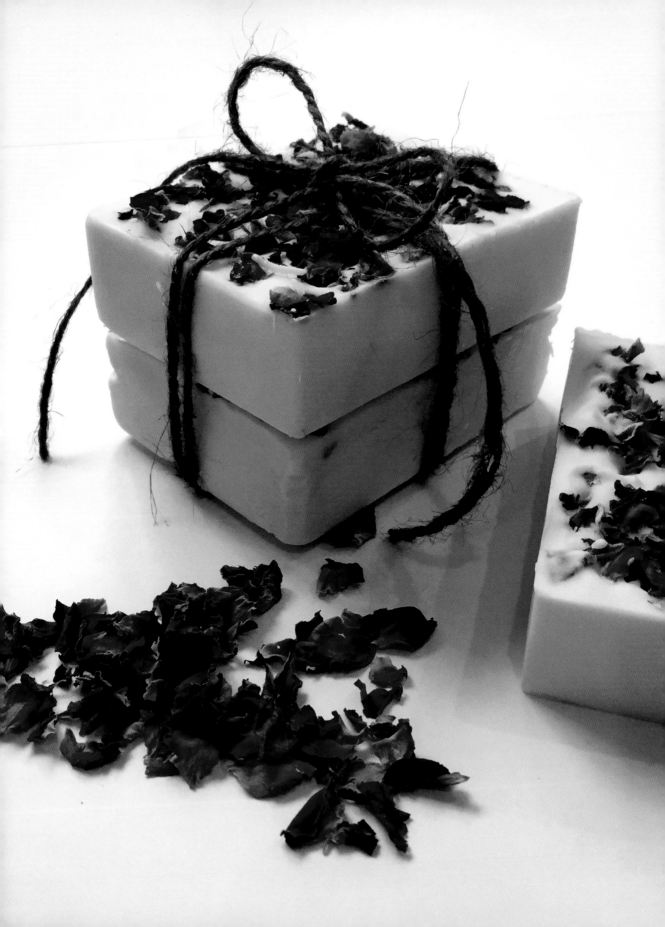

CHAPTER TWELVE

MAKE YOUR OWN SOAP

YOU DON'T HAVE TO CREATE SOAP FROM SCRATCH IF YOU WANT A HOMEMADE PRODUCT. YOU CAN USE SOAP FLAKES INSTEAD. BUT IF YOU WANT TO TRY MAKING IT FROM THE BEGINNING, PERHAPS FOR THE FUN OF IT, HERE IS AN OUTLINE OF THE THEORY, THE PRACTICAL INSTRUCTIONS AND PLENTY OF SAMPLE RECIPES

SOAP

... is the first choice when it comes to removing dirt that contains oils and grease. Without soap, water is not able to remove greasy impurities, because fats are water repellent. They isolate themselves from the water immediately, even if they have been vigorously stirred together. In order for the water to dissolve greasy dirt, it needs an emulsifier. Something that really goes for the fat. Soap.

HISTORY OF SOAP

People already had an early version of soap 5,000 years ago. On the cuneiform tablets of the Sumerians, there is a kind of recipe for something that comes very close to today's soft soap. A short time later, the Egyptians immortalised the first real soap recipes on papyrus. Essential components of ancient Egyptian soaps were various fats or oils and the ashes of certain plants. It was customary to boil the soap. In the Roman thermal baths, visitors were given a piece of soap made from goat fat and wood ash as part of their entrance fee. These so-called 'Mattish Balls' were named after the city of Mattium, a centre of Roman soap production, and they must have been a rather rough and only mildly fragrant detergent. The fact that this soap was quite harsh to the skin did not bother the Romans. After cleansing, they re-oiled their bodies.

The ashes that turn fat into soap contain sodium carbonate ie 'washing soda'. It forms crystals and, when dissolved in water, caustic soda. The caustic soda (sodium hydroxide) reacts with oils and fats, even with oily and greasy dirt, to form soap. Soaps are solids that are formed from the reaction of the caustic soda solution and the fatty acids. The residual 'slime', the soaps, can be loosened from the water and rinsed away.

The ancient Egyptian principle of soap making has been maintained to this day with slight variations. Instead of the soda they derived from plant or wood ash, today we use sodium hydroxide solution (caustic soda) instead. If the quantity of ingredients is not calculated precisely, residues of the caustic soda solution may remain in the soap, which is not at all good for the skin. The caustic soda heats itself up to over 80 °C when it comes into contact with water and may even start spontaneously boiling, foaming and spraying. Getting splashes of boiling caustic soda on the skin or, worse, in the eye, is the kind of household accident you should absolutely avoid.

MAKING YOUR OWN SOAP FROM SCRATCH ///////////////////////////////

[For the more faint-hearted, see easy soap-making page 208]

Because soap boiling is not without its dangers, the necessary precautions are listed here before we start.

Safety glasses and rubber gloves are absolutely essential. A full apron or overall is recommended, ideally with sleeves that protect the skin on the arms. Closed shoes protect the skin on the feet from any splashes that land on the floor. You should put on this protective clothing before you start weighing caustic soda and fats or oils.

- When the caustic soda solution is dissolved in water, vapours are produced which should not be inhaled under any circumstances. When mixing the caustic soda, very good ventilation of the room is essential.

When handling the caustic soda solution, the following rules should be strictly followed:

- **The caustic soda is always added to the water, never the water poured over the caustic soda!**

- If the caustic soda solution is added to the melted fat or heated oil, it should be poured slowly and carefully through a sieve into the fat melt. In this way you can filter out the flakes that have not dissolved in water.

- If, despite all precautionary measures, splashes of caustic soda solution get onto your skin or even worse into your eyes, rinse immediately with plenty of water! Especially with splashes in the eyes, you must see a doctor immediately.

- Caustic soda solution can be neutralized by vinegar, so a bottle of vinegar should always be available for emergencies. Splashes on worktops can be wiped away. Promptly pour vinegar on any spillage then wipe it away with kitchen paper.

Caustic soda must not come into contact with aluminium or cast iron. **These materials are an absolute taboo in soap making.**
All containers should be made of stainless steel, glass or enamel, possibly also heat-resistant and alkali-resistant plastic.

If you are not manufacturing your soap according to a specific recipe, use an online soap calculator to calculate the exact amount of caustic soda solution required for the selected fats or oils and their quantity.

Fats and oils have a saponification number. It is of critical importance for the success of a soap. With their help you can, with precision, avoid the over-fatting of a soap and ensure that no unsaponified caustic soda remains in the finished product. Your aim is to achieve a minimal over-greasing of the soap: there must always be a little more grease than the caustic solution can saponify. That way you're always on the safe side.

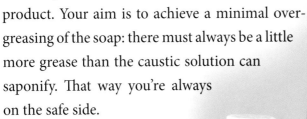

Coconut fat, for example, has the saponification number 0.183.

To saponify 100g coconut fat, you calculate:

100 x 0.183 = 18.3

It takes 18.3 grams of caustic soda solution (in the solid state, before dissolving in water) to completely saponify 100 grams of coconut fat.

As far as the amount of water needed to dissolve caustic soda is concerned, one can stick to an old soap maker rule of thumb: **two-thirds of fat quantity is needed to one-third water for the caustic soda**.

So if you want to saponify 90g of fat, you need 30g of water to dissolve the calculated amount of caustic soda. And as stated earlier: caustic soda is always added *to* the water, never the other way round!

Caustic soda for the production of soap should be bought in a specialist shop or online. It should be as pure as possible – 98 per cent pure is usual – and should not contain any additives. This is important because doctored caustic soda is sometimes sold as a drain cleaner in DIY stores.

The step-by-step instructions on the following pages are for the production of floral soap made from coconut fat and lard. Afterwards you will find a basic recipe for soap made from olive oil.

MAKE YOUR OWN FLOWER SOAPS

Cold process soap-making

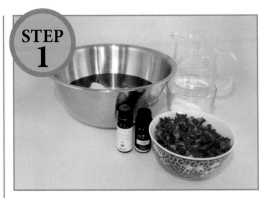

STEP 1

The ingredients: Fat (eg. coconut fat, lard etc), water, caustic soda, dried flowers, essential oil.

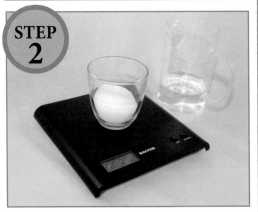

STEP 2

Weigh the ingredients exactly!

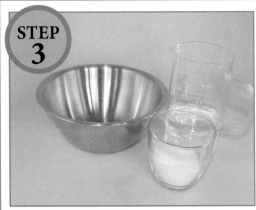

STEP 3

Stir the caustic soda slowly and carefully into the water.

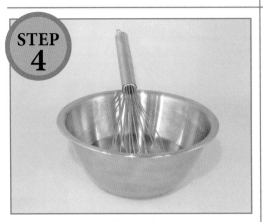

STEP 4

Mix well.

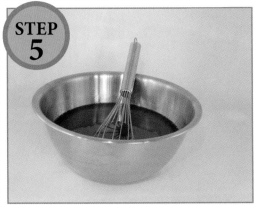

STEP 5

Melt the fat in a water bath.

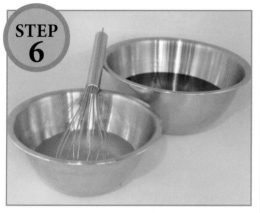

STEP 6

Pour the caustic soda slowly and carefully into the melted fat.

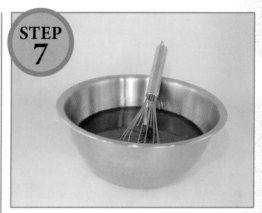

STEP 7

Carefully mix them together using a whisk.

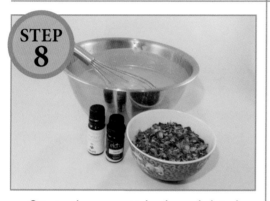

STEP 8

Stir in the essential oils and dried flowers once the mixture has cooled a bit.

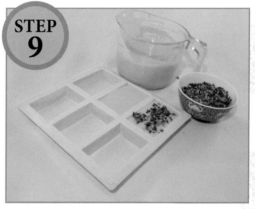

STEP 9

Pour the finished liquid soap into the moulds.

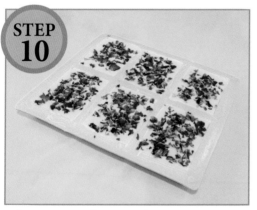

STEP 10

As soon as the soap has set, you can turn it out of the mould.

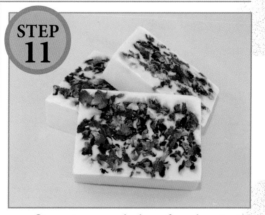

STEP 11

Store in a cool place for about 8 weeks to mature.

EQUIPMENT AND MATERIALS FOR THE SOAP FACTORY

Even if you already have all the equipment you need in your kitchen, any items that come into direct contact with the caustic soda solution should *only* be used to make soap. In this way, you avoid any traces getting into your foods. You need a large pan made of stainless steel or enamel (not aluminium!), a stirring rod (preferably made of glass), some measuring cups and a scale accurate to the gram (preferably a digital scale).

If you want to turn several different types of fats and oils into soap, you will need a hand blender or food processor to mix the oils or fats well during the melting process.

To shape the soap, you need soap moulds, either bought cheaply from a craft shop or cut by yourself from yoghurt pots, margarine bowls or similar food packaging. A dough scraper is useful to bring all the soap residues from the pan into the moulds.

The materials used to make a soap are fats or oils and caustic soda. That's all it takes. Basically you can use any fats, even old engine oil or deep-frying grease. However, since it is nearly impossible to determine the exact composition and therefore the saponification number for such fats, it is better not to touch them. Of course, oils and fats for soap production should be available at a reasonable price. But you don't have to compromise on quality.

In the following, some fats and oils are listed by saponification number, and are recommended for homemade soap production.

COCONUT FAT (saponification number 0.183) provides a hard soap with a weak foam. It should only be used to a maximum of 30 per cent in a fat mixture.

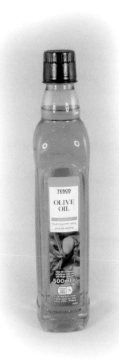

OLIVE OIL (saponification number 0.135) has created the famous Aleppo soap for centuries. It results in a mild soap, but without further fats as an addition it takes a very long time to solidify.

RAPESEED OIL (saponification number 0.135) is a very inexpensive but nevertheless high-quality domestic oil, which provides a mild soap for sensitive skin. However, a pure rapeseed oil soap forms very little foam.

SUNFLOWER OIL (saponification number 0.135)

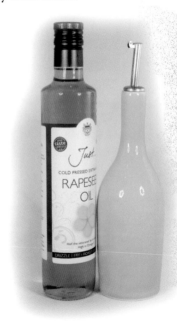

is inexpensive and produces a soft soap that does not form much foam. It should therefore be mixed with a proportion of a highly foaming fat, such as coconut fat.

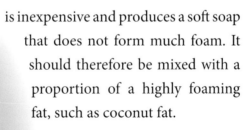

SAFFLOWER OIL (saponification number 0.136) is a skin caring oil with a high content of unsaturated fatty acids. However, safflower oil alone produces a very soft soap and should therefore be combined with hard fats.

PUMPKIN SEED OIL (saponification number 0.135) is quite expensive, but has a pleasantly nutty scent, which remains in the soap. The result is a mild, nourishing soap with a firm consistency.

LINSEED OIL (saponification number 0.134) makes the soap very soft and produces little foam. On its own it does not lead to satisfactory results, so it should be combined with other, more solid fats.

LARD (saponification number 0.140) gives the soap a good, firm consistency and a rich, stable foam. Soaps made from pure lard are bright white.

BASIC RECIPE FOR OLIVE OIL SOAP WITH LAVENDER FLOWERS

1000g olive oil
126g caustic soda
335g water (or distilled water if the water from the tap is too hard)
10g dried lavender heads
20 drops essential lavender oil

The ratio of olive oil to caustic soda in this recipe is deliberately slightly higher in order to moisturise the skin with the residual olive oil.

The carefully-measured water is placed in a pan (stainless steel or enamelled, never aluminium) or a caustic and heat-resistant bowl with a capacity of at least two litres. Slowly add the caustic soda and stir carefully. The resulting caustic solution heats up very quickly and can reach up to 80 °C. Stir until the caustic soda is clear again and let it cool down to about 40 to 45 °C.

It is important to add the caustic soda to the water and under no circumstances to pour the water over it.

In a second pan, heat the olive oil to the same temperature as the caustic soda solution and then pour the caustic soda liquid slowly into the oil, stirring constantly. This solution is stirred until it thickens, forming the soap melt. This takes about a quarter of an hour, and you should do it by hand – using a hand whisk or a wooden spoon – and not with a blender.

When the soap melt has an even consistency, you can either pour it into moulds and let it thicken into the soap. Or you can embellish it with lavender in this recipe. To do this, stir the dried lavender flowers and then the essential lavender oil evenly into the soap melt.

This soap melt is poured into moulds, covered and left to stand in a warm place for at least two days. In this time the saponification takes place and the soap develops a firm consistency. Once the soap is solid, it is removed from the mould and, if it is quite large, cut to the desired size in blocks. Before using the soap, it should be left to mature for about eight weeks. The bars of soap are placed on their narrow side so that they have as much surface contact as possible with the air.

From this basic recipe you can produce many different types of solid soaps. All you have to do is know the saponification numbers of the oils and fats used and calculate the **exact** amount of caustic soda required.

There is hardly any limit to creativity in soap making. For example, you can replace the water with a herbal decoction. Caustic soda in herbal decoction creates caustic soda solution in the same way as with water. Dried flowers can be stirred into the soap melt according to personal preference, and the soap can be coloured or marbled. If you stir some carrot juice into the finished soap melt, the soap takes on an orange colour. A brown soap is made with black coffee, cinnamon or cocoa. The scents matching the colour are added to the soap by adding the appropriate essential oils.

EASY SOAP FROM SOAP FLAKES

If you find the method of soap making described above too complicated, you can instead make your own soap creations from soap flakes. Soap flakes can be bought in bags or grated from solid curd soap or glycerine soap. This makes soap production as easy as can be:

- Put the required quantity of soap flakes in a bowl.

- Kneading continuously, add spoonfuls of water or herbal decoction until a thick dough is formed.

- Stir into this paste your dried flowers, herbs, essential oils or colouring agents such as carrot juice, coffee, cocoa or cinnamon, and also nourishing additives such as melted beeswax or dried, finely powdered propolis.

- Pour this thick soap melt into moulds and let it dry, preferably overnight, until it reaches a firm consistency. Then you can squeeze your soaps out of the moulds and let them dry for about two days.

INDEX

A

B

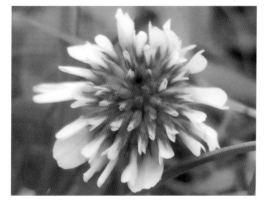

C

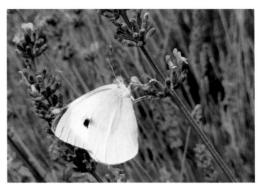

D

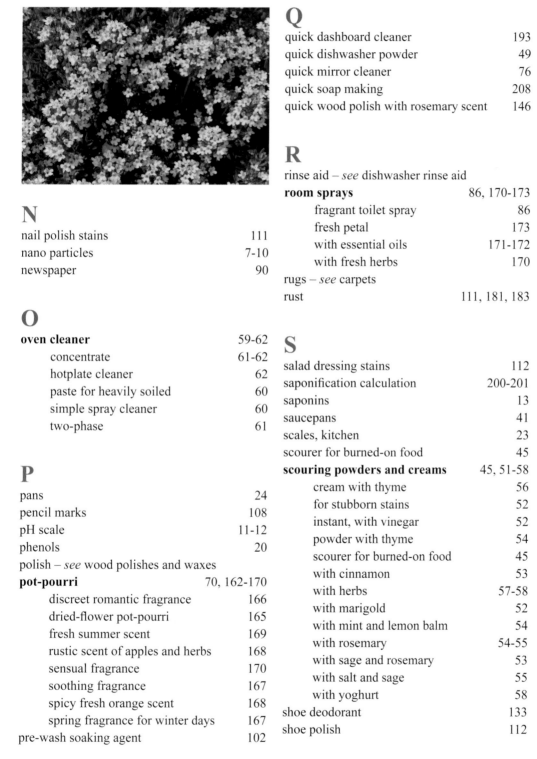

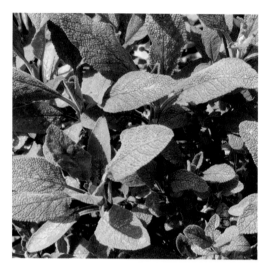

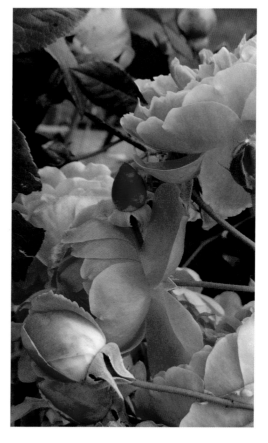

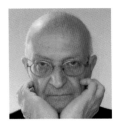